Tomorrow Never Comes

Tomorrow Never Comes

Buddy Young

iUniverse, Inc.
New York Lincoln Shanghai

Tomorrow Never Comes

iUniverse books may be ordered through booksellers or by contacting:

iUniverse
2021 Pine Lake Road, Suite 100
Lincoln, NE 68512
www.iuniverse.com
1-800-Authors (1-800-288-4677)

This is a true story, only the names have been changed to protect the privacy of my friends and associates. The only names that weren't changed were that of myself, my wife, and those diseased.

ISBN-13: 978-0-595-36293-6 (pbk)
ISBN-13: 978-0-595-80733-8 (ebk)
ISBN-10: 0-595-36293-1 (pbk)
ISBN-10: 0-595-80733-X (ebk)

Printed in the United States of America

This book is dedicated to my wonderful wife Sandy
So her memory will live forever.
I will love no other, forever, as I have loved her.

Contents

1

The Happiest Man Alive

I think I must have been the happiest man alive. I was able to retire early and we purchased our retirement home a year ago in Red Bluff, CA. When we woke up the very first morning we looked out of our sliding glass door and saw 13 deer and a flock of turkeys. It was exciting at first. Our home was new but didn't have any landscaping. The house is on an acre of land with probably 100 oak trees. My wife and I always did things our self, so we started the landscaping right away. Sandy would dig out the hard red clay soil that was on our land and have planting mix brought in. She would then plant her flowers and plants. She loved lavender and planted a lot of lavender plants. In the summer when the lavender would bloom it would smell so nice.

It gets hot in the summer so we would only work until noon, then we would come in and clean up and have lunch. Sandy would be very dirty from planting fruit trees and flowers and would have to take her clothes off and head straight for the shower. We loved working in the yard. I started building a fence to inclose our backyard because the deer would eat our flowers, plants and fruit trees. Sandy would be laying in bed at night and quite often see a deer looking in our sliding glass door at her. She would get up, open the door and scare them away.

Before I get into the tragedy that struck our family and how I dealt with it, let me introduce you to our families and our friends.

My name is Buddy Young, I'm 58 years old and I retired over a year ago after a successful career in retail management working for the same company for 36 years. I'm 6'1" tall and weigh 200 pounds. I have red hair, although it's kind of whitish now and I have a bald spot in the back of my head. I didn't need glasses until after I was 40 and I didn't need hearing aids until after my 55th. Birthday. I was an athlete as a youth and even coached 7th. And 8th Grade basketball some years ago. My favorite pastime is playing golf, and working around the house.

My wife of 35 years was Sandy, a wonderful, generous and kind woman who always went out of her way to care for other people. She also cared very much for the special people in her life. She was a good person, wife, mother and grand-mother. She was 4'11" tall and I could put my arms straight out and twirl around and never hit her head. Sandy had dark brown hair and she always kept it pretty short because it is curly. Lately she has let her hair grow long. I didn't know why and she never told me but I would find out why later.

Sandy was very creative, imaginative and quite a good interior decorator. Her friends would always ask her for advice. She watched decorating shows all the time, and sometimes asks me to watch one of the shows with her. On some of the shows they would have something on that Sandy had done.

I would say, "they copied your idea."

Sandy would say, "no. That's been around awhile."

Sandy collected all of the paint samples the store had and kept them in a file for reference.

She would pin them on the wall and look at them for several days until she was satisfied that she found the right color. After painting the living room in our retirement home, Sandy decided that it was the wrong color so she had it tinted a little different and I painted again. Sandy said that the color still wasn't right so I painted a third time. I thought it looked ok to me the first two times I painted it, Sandy had to have it just the right color. I wouldn't know it at the time but Sandy always had a vision what the room would look like after it was decorated and I have to admit, she was always right.

Sandy loved to work in her garden. She once told me while working in her garden, "I love it when I have more work than I can do." She planted lots of trees and flowers and she would talk to them. She would work all day in her garden repotting plants and starting new ones off of cuttings.

Sandy loved birdwatching. She had several books on birds and had binoculars in every room. She had me build several bird houses and hook them to the trees outside. Sandy also hung bird feeders outside to attract different species of birds. When she saw a bird that she didn't know, she would get out her books and look it up. Sandy loved to lay in bed when she woke up in the morning and watch the birds.

Sandy was a great cook and loved to cook gourmet dinners and would do so when we would have friends or family over. On one thanksgiving we had my brothers, their family's, and my mother over for dinner. My mother was in a wheel chair then and when she saw a metal figurine of a black cat in the yard, she said, "Sidney, they let you out." Sidney is the only male and the oldest of our four cats. Mom's eyesight was failing her. She once told me that she memorized where all the stop signs were in the town she lived in. Of course we wouldn't let her drive anymore after that.

Sandy cooked for three days. I remember we had thirteen different deserts. We had turkey, stuffing, mashed potatoes, yams, asparagus, green beans, cranberry sauce, and dinner rolls. Sandy fixed other things too but I can't remember all of them. My brother Kermit has six children so we sent most of the leftovers home with him. She wanted to make it special for my side of the family, and she did. I think it was the most extravagant meal she ever cooked. It was an event to remember.

I met Sandy in the grocery store I worked in. One day the boss hired this pretty girl and I didn't pay much attention to her at first. She lived across the street from me and would come over and tell me when she had done something good a work. She was so excited to have done well. After some time I started dating Sandy and we were married on February 5, 1970. When we got married we didn't have any money or furniture just like most people. We had a cantaloupe crate for a coffee table and friends of ours gave us an old sofa that folded down flat. We slept on that sofa until we could afford a bed. The sofa had a hole where the crease was and I would wake up at night and my leg would be stuck down that hole. It also had a broken spring that would poke me in the rear at night. We bought a used refrigerator at a second hand store for $35 and after a while we bought a sleigh bed at a second hand store for $7. Those days when we were starting out had some memorable times.

We moved six times throughout my career and each time it gave Sandy another chance to decorate our new house. All the moves were hard on Sandy though because each time we moved she had to find a new job. Sandy was, however, very supportive of my career.

We have two children and three grandchildren. Our son Michael (born November 23,1968) is in law enforcement. After graduating from high school Michael joined the air force and served in Korea. He was fortunate enough to see some of the Olympic games while he was over there. I think he got to see the men's volleyball finals. He collects hockey memorabilia. He has hockey sticks, jerseys, and lots and lots of cards and autographs. Michael went to several San Jose Sharks hockey games each year and took me to one year before last. He was disappointed that the contract negotiations stalled this year because he couldn't see any games. He's a sports nut like his Dad. Michael's wife, Lona is a wonderful person. They have three children, two daughters and a son. Marie, Candy, and Hugh. Candy and Marie are in high school now and Candy played some basketball and Marie is a cheerleader. We get to see her often because she goes to cheerleading competitions in Sacramento and her and her family stay with us on their way. Our home is ½ way from their home to the competition so it's a good stopping off and resting place. Our beautiful daughter Nicole was born on March 22,1971 and she is in the law profession. Nicole is still going to college and is scheduled to graduate next spring. Sandy was so much looking forward to going to Nicole's graduation. Nicole has beautiful, long, curly brown hair. I think she could have been a hair model.

We played a lot of games with our children when they were young, board games, card games, and dice games. When we took Nicole to register for kindergarten the teacher asked Nicole if she could count. Nicole said "yes I can, two, three, four, five, six, seven, eight, nine, ten, jack, queen, king, ace. Nicole could add any numbers up to six plus six. Of course six was the highest number on a die.

I have three brothers and a sister and I'm the shortest of all my brothers. My oldest brother Bill was the first born, then came me seventeen months later. My sister Carmen is eleven years younger than I am. Then a year later Lawrence was born and finally Kermit. It was like my parents had two families because Bill and I were grown and gone from home before my sister and two younger brothers grew up. Because of the age difference I was closer to Bill but as we grew older I became closer to my two younger brothers. I am very close to my sister now, we keep in touch all the time and visit each other when we can. All my brothers have red hair and Carmen is the only one who is not red headed, she has brown hair.

My older brother Bill died eight years ago of heart failure. Bill was a fantastic high school and junior college basketball player. Bill was also an all star basketball player in the army. He received many scholarship offers while he was in the army. One of his scholarship offers was to St. Bonaventure and he could have played with Bob Lanier but he didn't take advantage of any of his scholarship offers. Bill was also an avid fisherman. The only time I would ever go fishing was when I visited my brother, Bill. Bill would always catch twice as many fish as all the other people combined.

My sister Carmen lives in Australia and has one daughter, Karen, who moved back to the states a couple of years ago. Karen is now 23 and living with her father and going to college. Carmen loves it in Australia and I don't think she will ever move back to the states, although I've been trying to talk her into it.

In 1991 when we lived in Ukiah, my sister Carmen came to visit. She had her brother in law, John with her. When I answered the door, John had an Australian hat on and I said," I like your hat. He took the hat off his head and put it on mine. I then looked in my closet for something to give him. I found a warm up suit that was red, white and blue and it had U S A on the back in big red letters, so I gave that to him. John was excited to have it and when he got back home he showed it to all of his friends.

Carmen and I thought it would be a good idea to have all of our family come to my house for a reunion. Mom lived with us at the time so we didn't have to call her. My father passed away some 20 years earlier. We called my brothers and persuaded them to come to my house for the weekend. My older brother, Bill was hard to get a hold of but we finally tracked him down and talked him into coming for the weekend. We had a really good time and a great visit. At night we would sit around the living room and talk about the good old days and out of the corner of my eye I could see my mother taking it all in and smiling. She was happy to have all of her family together. My younger brother Kermit, his wife, and three boys came. His daughters were not born at that time. It was around Christmas time and Sandy took the three boys to the shoe store where she worked and bought them all new tennis shoes. When she came home with the boys, one of them told his father "dad aunt Sandy has a plastic card that turns into money, we have to get one of those." We had a good laugh about that.

In 2000 Carmen was going through a divorce and wanted me to go to Australia and be with her for a while. I planned the trip to stay in Australia for ten days and the flight over was very comfortable. The plane was less than half full and some people laid on the five seats in the middle and slept. Of course we crossed the international date line and when I arrived in Australia it was two days later. The time difference between California and Sidney is eighteen hours. If it is 9:00 A.M. on Friday in California, it's 5:00 A.M. Saturday in Sidney. If we are on daylight savings time the difference is seventeen hours. On the way to Australia we had to fill out a card and questionnaire if the passengers had anything to declare. One of the questions was, "do you have any drugs?" I had prescriptions with me so I checked yes. At customs the man asked me if the drugs were prescriptions prescribed by a doctor and I said "yes". So he let me go on through while they were searching other people's baggage. I thought to myself "when you travel, you should always declare something, that way maybe you wont be detained." There were a lot of signs at customs about mad cow disease. If any of the passengers were coming from London, they wanted to know about it.

Carmen raises cutting horses and she took me to a competition. Carmen took two of her horses and won first and third places. While we were at the competition, I went to get something to eat, and ordered a sausage sandwich. What I got was what looked like a farmer brown sausage on a piece of bread with butter on it. Butter was used a lot because mayonnaise was rare in Australia. Then I went to another stand and ordered a strawberry milkshake. Carmen was talking to a friend when I ordered and came over to me while I was waiting for it. She asked me what I ordered and I told her a strawberry milkshake. She said, "you didn't, did you."

I said, "yes, why?"

She said, "they're different over here, you have to tell them to make it really thick."

When I got the milkshake it was watery like strawberry flavored milk. At least I learned how to order a milk shake.

I did something while visiting Carmen that I haven't done in twenty years. We rode horses every day. I told Carmen to give me a gentle horse to ride as I was a novice. She said, "you can ride Rose." Rose is an older mare and very gentle, but well trained. Rose was perfect for me to ride. We would go round up the cattle every day and bring them into the pen so Carmen could practice with her cutting horses. Rose knew just what to do, if one of the cows would start to wander off, she would just go to the side of the cow and guide it back to the right direction, all I had to do was hang on. Like I said it was new to me and I woke up each morning with a sore butt.

Carmen lives in a small town in New South Wales called Tumut. Tumut is about a five hour drive inland from Sydney. Carmen would take me out sightseeing every day and I got to see a kangaroo and a lot of other wildlife native to Australia. Once when we stopped for gas I offered Carmen $35 for a tank of gas. She wouldn't take any money and just laughed.

I said," what are you laughing about?"

Carmen said, "gas is ninety nine cents a liter over here and it takes $100 to fill my tank." That would equate to $3.75 a gallon. Of course that was Australian money and I got almost two Australian dollars for one American dollar.

In our travels I saw what looked like very small man made lakes and asked Carmen, "what are those for."

Carmen said, "they're called dams. In the summer, the water is scarce so they have to build dams so the animals have water. There are people who specialize in building the dams and know just where to put them."

I asked Carmen, "I notice that all the cars and trucks over here have bars on the front, what are those for?"

Carmen said, "those are to protect your car from the kangaroos, they jump in front of cars and it's like hitting a cow."

We went to dinner one night with friends of hers, Steve and Sara, and it lasted four hours. Needless to say that dinner was a wonderful event. Steve and Sara owned a jewelry store and I bought my granddaughter, Mary, a charm bracelet and some charms. All of the charms were of Australian things. The only charm I remember was of a kangaroo. On the way to the jewelry store. I started to J walk and Carmen grabbed me by the arm and said, "Bud, if you cross the street here you are fair game, a driver might run over you. If you cross the street at a crosswalk, then you can cross anytime you want. The cars have to stop for you."

The people in Australia were friendly and nice. A lot of Carmen's friends were very interested in what I had to say about the comparison between the United Sates and Australia.

Carmen and I were invited to dinner by another one of her friends, Carmelita. Carmen told me that Carmelita claimed to be a witch. Not a witch in the terms that we use today, but a real witch. There were a lot of people there and Carmelita barbequed some sausages for dinner. Carmelita had some land cleared and the trees piled up in a huge pile. After dark that night she set the pile of trees and brush on fire. The bonfire was close to some live trees and I thought they were going to catch fire. I couldn't help telling some of the people that if it was in the States, they would have to clear at least ten feet around the bonfire, get a permit, and have water available in case the fire got out of control.

At the dinner party there were three girls about eleven or twelve years old that were very interested in talking to me. I told them "in the states we drive on the right side of the road, over here you drive on the left side of the road. In the states the highway signs say yield and over here they say give way." I had a lot of other comparisons that I can't remember now but the girls were laughing and laughing at my stories.

We went to dinner at another one of Carmen's friends house and Carmen and I were going to cook taco's for them. The friend, Charlotte, and her husband Jeff, have a nineteen year old son, Mike. It was hard for us to find some of the ingredients for the taco's. Tortillas and olives were hard to find in the stores. We couldn't find canned olives in any of the stores, but we finally found tortillas in one store and olives in a deli. After dinner I was talking to Mike and told him that the only sports on T.V. was Cricket, and I asked him to explain the game to me. Mike said the pitcher had to keep his arm straight by rule and that some pitchers could throw up to 100 miles an hour. Mike said that there was a stick behind the batter and the pitcher tries to hit the stick, if he does the batter is out. Mike went on to explain that there is a runner on first when the batter is at bat. When the batter hits the ball, the runner on first runs home and the batter runs to first. That is scored as one run. The batter has a choice whether to run or not.

When a batter hits a home run it counts as four runs. I guess that explains why the scores are so high.

My ten day visit came to an end and Carmen drove me to the airport. I had a three hour wait for my flight out of Sydney so I bought gifts for everyone back home. I wondered around the airport shops and I bought a scarf for Sandy, gifts for my mother in law and the neighbor kids. I also bought a polo shirt for me that said Australia on it.

The metric system is used in Australia. When the weather man gave the temperature it was in Celsius so I had to multiply by nine and divide by five and add thirty two so I could figure out how hot it was. The produce and meat in the grocery stores were sold by the Kilogram. I noticed the meat department had a large display of lamb and a small display of beef. Australia is famous for it's lamb and it is sold in the United States.

When I left Sydney to come home it was noon and when I arrived home it was 9:00 A.M. on the same day so I got home, by the clock, before I left even though it was a fifteen hour flight. On the flight home from Australia the plane was completely full and the guy's seat in front of me seemed like it was only inches from my face. It was very uncomfortable. I couldn't sleep and when I got home I was so tired that I went straight to bed and slept for several hours. Then I got up and ate dinner and it was time for bed. It took me three days to get over the jet lag.

The only regret I have is that I didn't spend a day sightseeing in Sydney. Sydney is the capitol of New South Wales and is Australia's oldest European settlement. I think I would like to go back someday.

My little brother Lawrence (I should say younger not little because he is 6'6" tall) was disabled after losing his right leg below the knee in a mill accident. He has a prosthesis and it doesn't keep him from doing the things he wants to do. I always admired him for that. Lawrence is divorced and has two children. Laura, his daughter is married and has children or her own. Lawrence also has a son, Kile.

My youngest brother Kermit, also 6'6", is employed by an armored car company. Kermit is married to Darby and has six children, three boys and three girls. Bob is the oldest followed by Charles and Tommy. The three girls are Katie, Andrea, and Myrna. All of my brothers and sister were athletic when we were younger. Kermit played semi pro baseball in Canada, he was a pitcher. All my brothers played basketball in high school.

My wife, Sandy has four brothers and a sister. Sandy's oldest brother, Lark lives in Wyoming and owns a fish and chip's restaurant. He used to be a commercial fisherman like his father William, but the ocean being so dangerous, he looked for another trade. Lark was the entrepreneur of the family.

Her brother Daniel, is still a commercial fisherman and lives in California. Sandy's brother Sparky used to be a commercial fisherman but now is a cabinet maker. Sparky and his wife Melissa are getting a divorce. Sparky is having a tough time because he is going through Sandy's illness as well as a divorce. Sparky has two daughters, Sheila is in high school and is a straight A student, Sophie is only seven and is having a tough time adjusting to her parents separation.

Sandy's brother Charles and his wife Tara are both school teachers. Charles used to be a commercial fisherman, but sold his boats and Charles and his wife, Tara, went back to college. They both became teachers. Charles and Tara have three boys, Troy the oldest has graduated from high school and moved away from home, Tommy and Chuck still live at home and the boys like their father, love to hunt and fish. They are also big sports nuts.

Sandy's youngest brother, Tommy lost his life in a boating accident on the ocean years ago. I think this played a large part in three of the other brothers seeking new occupations.

Sandy's sister, Dana is divorced and lives in the same town in California as we do. Dana has two grown sons. Alfred is an accountant and a pilot. He just opened his first Quisno's sandwich franchise in southern California. It looks like he will be a successful business man. Lone is an ex-marine and wholesales diving gear.

My two best friends are Lane Yeperson and Lance Butterman. I met Lane at work when I worked in Burney and we became friends. He went though a divorce and he thought he was the bad guy. I supported my friend Lane and it turned out that he was the good guy. I won't go through the details here to protect the privacy of those involved, after all this is a true story. Lane has curly brown hair and he has a bigger bald spot in the back of his head than I do. Lane and I are both sports nuts so we have a lot in common. Lane even does some side work as a referee. Lane was remarried to a wonderful woman named Clair. Lane loved to cook and Clair didn't like to, so they have an agreement, Lane would cook and she would clean up. Lane cooks with so much love that he needs big pots and pans to cook in. Clair is a Berkley grad and is an excellent graphic designer.

One day when I was on vacation, Lane called me at home, he had a problem at the store. I got mad because someone would call me while I was on vacation, but went to the store to sort out the problem. Lane was in tears when I got there and that's when I realized what a sensitive person he was. I sorted out the problem, and it wasn't hard at all. Later I was transferred to Redding and when I had an opening Lane transferred there to be my produce manager.

I met Lance while I was working in Redding. He worked with me at the store and we became friends and played a lot of golf together. Lance retired two years before I did and my brother Lawrence played golf with Lance and I. Lawrence said that the golf was one of his favorite memories. Lance's wife was Eloise and she worked in city government. While we were both still working, we planned a trip to Las Vegas. Our wives had not met at that time and we were a little worried if they would get along with each other. We had to laugh about that after they got to know each other because they became close friends. Sandy and Eloise would go shopping while Lance and I would go play golf. We would always get home before the girls so we knew they were having a good time, after all it was their favorite activity.

After I was transferred to Rocklin Lance and Eloise would come and visit us. Eloise liked that because there was good shopping there. Once when they came to visit, they no more got in the door and the girls looked at each other and almost at the same time said, "are you ready to go?." The girls didn't even unpack their bags, they just took off out the door because they couldn't wait to go shopping. Lance and I just looked at each other and shrugged our shoulders. We sat down and watched a professional basketball game. Our favorite team, the Kings were playing so we enjoyed the game.

Sandy worked for a man in Burney, we also became friends with him and his family. His name is George. George is a handsome man with dark hair, and is a good employer for Sandy. His wife's name is Candy and they have a daughter, Briana. Candy is a tall pretty woman with blond hair. Briana also has blond hair and is a pretty girl. Sandy always thought of Briana as another granddaughter. George owned two gas station, convenience stores and Sandy would drive back and forth and work at both of them. When I retired and we moved to Red Bluff, George helped us move.

2

A Hospital Stay

In May 2004 Sandy had a cap fall off her tooth and went to the dentist to have it put back on. She started feeling bad after that, and after a couple of weeks she came to me and said, "Buddy, I'm sick." It was time to go to the doctor. It was a weekend so we had to go to the emergency room at the hospital. Her gums were swollen and bleeding. The doctor at the emergency room thought Sandy had a dental infection and gave her a prescription for an antibiotic.

Another week went by and Sandy wasn't feeling any better, she was actually feeling worse, Her eye's were baggy and swollen, her gums were swollen and bleeding, and her neck was swollen. We went to see Sandy's doctor, doctor Chen, she is a thin, pleasant woman, with long dark hair. I went in the room to meet doctor Chen because I had a different doctor. Doctor Chen greeted me, shook my hand, and introduced herself. Doctor Chen was very pleasant, soft spoken, and gave me the impression that she really cared about her patients. Sandy told me later that doctor Chen was the best doctor she ever had and she tried to get me to switch doctors. Doctor Chen took a blood test and told Sandy to go to the hospital over the weekend and have another blood test done. She wanted to see if the white blood counts were going in the right direction. When a person has an infection, the white blood cells are what fight's the infection, so they naturally go up.

The upcoming weekend was Memorial day weekend so we went into the hospital on Sunday to have the blood work done. Doctor Chen had made all the arrangement and they were waiting for us. Sandy could hardly wait until Tuesday so she could see her doctor again, she was getting worse.

I had made plans a week prior to have some friends over to help he put in my putting green. I told Sandy that I would cancel the plans to put in the putting green and reschedule them for later. Sandy told me not to cancel the plans, but to go ahead and get the putting green put in. She said, "the putting green is in my landscaping plans." I think she was just as anxious as I was to get the job completed.

My friend Lane Yeperson brought his cousin Jim along with him to help. Jim was a tall thin man who had lost sight in one eye. He was a contractor so he knew how to do lots of things but I should have picked someone with two good eyes to help me seem the synthetic turf. I think Jim came along because he was single and wanted to meet Sandy's sister, Dana, who was also single. She was coming to help with the putting green. Lane's wife Clair came along and visited a little with Sandy, although Sandy spent some of the time in bed. Lance Butterman also came to help that day, along with my little brother Lawrence. I had the sub base already prepared and the cup holes already cut. I used decomposed granite for the sub base and the putting green was rather large, more than a thousand square feet. After we laid the carpet and seamed it we put 2000 pounds of sand on top so that when we would putt the ball would roll just on the tips of the fibers. It took us all day and when we finished we all took turns putting.

Finally Tuesday rolled around and we got up, had something to eat and went straight to the doctor's office. When we checked in, we asked to see the nurse. The nurse told us that there were no appointments until 11:20 and the doctor didn't get there until 9:00. Sandy said to the nurse, "I'm not leaving, I'm sick and I have to lie down." The nurse then showed Sandy to a room where she could lay down and wait for the doctor. Sandy didn't want me to go with her so I stayed in the waiting room and read the paper.

I thought we were going to be picking up a different antibiotic because the first one didn't work. Boy was I wrong. Sandy came out of the doctors office about 9:20. The doctor must have seen her first when she found out that Sandy was there, I knew the doctor was expecting her.

I asked Sandy, "what did the doctor say"

And Sandy said, "I'm supposed to go home and pack a bag. They think I have Leukemia. We're supposed to go to Redding to doctor Flag's office. They're waiting for us."

I was silent for a moment. I was in shock. I asked Sandy what she had to pack a bag for and she said, "incase they have to admit me to the hospital."

We drove home and sandy packed all of her pajamas, some under ware, and some slippers. Sandy hated those open backed hospital gowns. On the 30 minute drive to Redding neither one of us said too much, I think we were still in shock and didn't know what to think. I was very scared and somewhat in a daze but I didn't want Sandy to see how scared I was. I was also very nervous and didn't know what to say, I fiddled with the radio a lot and ran my hand through my hair. Sandy was silent the whole trip, she just stared straight ahead. The drive seemed to take hours.

When we arrived at the doctors office they were indeed waiting for us but the doctor wouldn't be there for another 10 minutes. After a short wait in the waiting room the nurse showed us to a room and the doctor came in shortly after that. Doctor Cambridge was very kind and tried to comfort us. He was a little heavy set with short dark hair. He appeared to be in his mid 40s. And wore a blue shirt with blue dockers. I found out later that he was a two-time cancer survivor. Later I saw his picture on the wall of the hospital. He was the chief of staff. Doctor Cambridge told us that Sandy had Leukemia and wanted to admit her to the hospital right away. I asked doctor Cambridge, "how do you know it's Leukemia?" The doctor said, "by the blood counts, the white blood count is high." He said, "I'm 99% sure, we need to do a bone marrow biopsy and send it to the lab to confirm that and to tell us what type of Leukemia it is. We need to know what type it is so we can administer the correct treatment." I asked doctor Cambridge, "when do we do the biopsy." He said, "I do it right here in my office." The doctor left the room to get his supplies and while he was gone I started to cry. Sandy said to me, "Buddy I need you to be strong now." I said, "it's not fair." The doctor came back a few minutes later assured us that he would take good care of Sandy. I asked the doctor how long the hospital stay would be and he said about a month. I held her hand as he did the bone marrow biopsy. Then he admitted Sandy to the hospital.

I stayed in the hospital with my wife until 10:00 that night and then drove home to sleep. On the way home my mind was racing, thinking about the events of the day. I was in a daze. I would just stare at the road and when I got home I couldn't remember driving home.

The next day before I went back to the hospital to visit Sandy, I called our children, Michael and Nicole. They were both devastated. It's hard to know exactly what their reaction was as I couldn't see their faces, however as I called each of them and told them of the bad news, there was silence on the phone for what seemed like quite a while. Both of the kids wanted to come and see their mother right away and I told them to wait until she got out of the hospital and was feeling better.

I was a manager during my career and was used to being in charge, solving problems and being a counselor for my employees, but now I was helpless. There was nothing I could do. I had to trust the doctors and their expertise in their field. I felt tired, I was completely wore out. I didn't have any trouble sleeping that night because I thought that everything would be alright.

The doctor used so many medical terms when he was talking to us that we became confused. The following information is from information supplied by the doctors.

- Chemotherapy is the use of various anticancer drugs to destroy the growth of cancer cells. Chemotherapy can consist of one drug or a group of drugs that work together. Usually, in the bone marrow transplant setting, a combination of drugs is used. Some chemotherapy can be orally (in a pill form), but most are given intravenously (through the central line).

- Bone marrow is a soft spongy tissue found inside the bones. When withdrawn form the bone, it looks just like blood. Its main function is to make blood cells, mainly red blood cells, white blood cells, and platelets. Every type of blood cell in the marrow begins as a stem cell. Without bone marrow and the disease-fighting blood cells it produces, your immune function will be weakened and you will not have a good defense against most common infections.

- Leukemia is a malignant disease (cancer) that originates in a cell in the marrow. It is characterized by the uncontrolled growth of developing marrow cells.

- Leukemia is a rapidly progressing disease that results in the accumulation of immature, functionless cells in the marrow and blood. The marrow often can no longer produce enough normal red and white blood cells and platelets.

- The term blood count refers to the number of blood cells circulating in your blood stream. There are three main types of cells, white blood cells, red blood cells, and platelets.

- White blood cells are responsible for fighting infection. These include neutrophils and lymphocytes. You are more susceptible to infection, and will be less resistant to illness when there is a decrease in the production of white blood cells. Neutrophils are responsible for fighting mostly bacterial and fungal infections. Lymphocytes are responsible for fighting viruses and for forming antibodies that will attack infectious organisms. A decrease in the number of neutrophils is called neutropenia.

- Red blood cells carry oxygen from the lungs throughout the body. The hematocrit means the percentage of blood that contains red blood cells. The hemoglobin is the part of the red blood cells that carries oxygen. Anemia occurs when there are not enough red blood cells in the blood. Some symptoms of anemia are shortness of breath, weakness, fatigue, dizziness, headache, and irritability.

- Platelets help control bleeding. When you cut yourself, the platelets form a clot to stop the bleeding. Some symptoms of low platelets are petechiae (small red dots on the skin) easy bruising, and bleeding from the gums or nose. A low platelet count is called thrombocytopenia.

The next day I visited my wife in the hospital. The surgical team put in a Groshong. A Groshong is a central venous catheter. (A special tube that is surgically inserted into a large vein near the heart and exits from the chest near the neck. The catheter allows medications, fluids, or blood products to be given and blood samples taken.

The lab tests came back the next day and confirmed that Sandy had A.M.L. (Acute Myeloid Leukemia) type five. The doctor started the chemotherapy (a treatment of cancer with drugs) and it was to last for six days. At first I visited Sandy in the hospital every day and when she started to feel better she told me that I didn't need to come every day so I started to visit her every other day.

Sandy's brother Charles came to the hospital to visit Sandy and she had him cut off all of her hair before it fell out. She then braided her hair and put it in an envelope. She addressed it to "locks of love" or "locks for love". That was the first time I knew why she was growing her hair so long. So she could send it to an organization for a child who needed a wig.

As I mentioned Sandy loved to garden and she watered all of her plants and trees by hand. I took over the chore and it took me four hours every other day because it was so hot. When I would visit Sandy in the hospital she would always ask me if I watered her plants and flowers and I would say, "I watered them yesterday." she would say, "you better water them again today, it's pretty hot out there." She was worried that I wouldn't take proper care of her plants and flowers, So I would go home and water again.

Once a week Clair would water for me so I could be at the hospital with my wife.

I kept busy while Sandy was in the hospital putting in a drip system. My friend Lance and my brother Lawrence came to help me get started. I purchased all the materials and had them ready when they arrived. I didn't put them on a timer. I connected them to faucets. We installed two small lines and then spent some time putting on my new putting green. I then drove to the hospital to be with Sandy for the rest of the day.

I worked on the drip system a little bit each day while Sandy was in the hospital. I wanted Sandy to be proud of me when she got home.

After 10 days or so Sandy started to feel like her old self again and I took her yarn to her so she could crochet baby blankets. A vision that has stuck in my mind was when I went to see my wonderful wife in the hospital she would be crocheting and when she saw me come through the door she smiled and put her crocheting down, got up out of her chair and gave me a big hug and a kiss. She was happy to see me and I was happy to see her.

Unfortunately chemotherapy kills good cells as well as cancer cells, so when Sandy's blood counts were too low she received blood transfusions and platelets. The nurses took blood every day to send to the lab and check her blood counts. It only took about an hour for the results to come back, so if Sandy needed blood or medications, they could start them right away.

After Sandy's body started to recover and make its own red and white blood cells and platelets, Sandy would be released from the hospital to go home and recover for a month. She was in the hospital for three weeks and was released on June 22, 2004, her 55th. Birthday. Doctor Cambridge told us that Sandy was a good candidate for a stem cell transplant because she was young and other wise in good health. Sandy told the doctor that she wanted to be cured so doctor Cambridge said he would set up an appointment for us at the University of California at San Francisco (U.C.S.F.), By July 4. The doctor's office called a week later and told us that they contacted the University of San Francisco and that they would be calling us with a date and time for our appointment.

We have four cats and Sandy loved them dearly and they loved Sandy. After I brought Sandy home from the hospital, Sandy didn't have an empty lap for days. She would sit in her favorite chair and crochet baby blankets and the cats would take turns in her lap. Sandy loved every minute of it.

Oh how our lives were about to change.

3

An Appointment

We spent the next month at home while Sandy's body recovered from the chemotherapy. Since chemotherapy kills all or most of the white blood cells, the doctor told us that Sandy would be susceptible to infection and it would take a year before she could work in her garden. He also told us to be very careful about being around people with coughs and colds. He also told us to be careful around children. Children carry a lot of germs and seem to be sniffling a lot of the time.

The doctors left the Groshong line in just incase it had to be used at a later date. During our month at home Sandy felt really good and resumed her household chores. I tried to help but she told me that she could do it.

I kept myself so busy while Sandy was in the hospital that I continued after she got home. One day while I was working outside on the drip system and Sandy called me for dinner and after dinner, I went back outside to work some more. Sandy was a little surprised that I was going nonstop. She could, however, still water her garden. All she had to do was turn on the faucet and then turn it off again when the watering was done. I think she enjoyed being able to still be involved in the care of her plants, trees and flowers.

We had to go back to the hospital every Friday so the nurse could flush the Groshong line to keep it from plugging up. On Friday, July 10, We got up and drove to the hospital to have Sandy's line flushed. On the way home Sandy started to feel sick. We continued home but Sandy got worse, so Sandy called the doctor and described what she was feeling. The doctor (doctor Flag this time) told us to go to the emergency room and he would arrange for direct admittance to the hospital. Doctor Flag ordered a blood test so they could determine what was wrong. The test indicated that Sandy had a staff infection. Doctor Flag ordered Vancomycin intravenously to treat the infection. The Doctor told us that Vancomycin is very effective against a staff infection and the nurses told us that it was used as an antibiotic when nothing else worked.

I looked Vancomycin up on the internet and found the following information:

- Vancomycin has become known as one of the most potent antistaphylococcal agents.

- Vancomycin is bactericidal and appears to exert its effect by binding to the precursor units of bacterial cell walls, inhibiting their syntheses. This binding occurs at a different site of action from that of penicillin. The net result is an alteration of mechanism of action.

- Resistance to Vancomycin is uncommon, although it has been reported in strains of group D Streptococcus.

Sandy was sent home after three days in the hospital and we were set up with home health care. Sandy was set up with a pump to administer the Vancomycin for another week or 10 days through her central venous catheter.

When the Vancomycin treatment was complete Sandy developed a whole body red rash. She called the doctor and he made an appointment for us to see a dermatologist. Sandy had a reaction to the Vancomycin and the dermatologist prescribed something for Sandy. Then we had another doctor's appointment for another bone marrow biopsy. The doctor wanted to see if the cancer was back or Sandy was still in remission. Afterwards we met with the doctor and he said there was no leukemia. Sandy was still in remission. Great news!

The oncology/hematology center at the University of California at San Francisco did call and we had an appointment on July 23, At 1:00P.M.

While we were waiting for our appointment in San Francisco, Sandy spent the time recovering from the chemotherapy.

4

Sidney and the Bear Dogs

It's amazing what races through a persons mind when his/her life is so dramatically changed and death is a possible outcome. I thought of everything in my past, even our four precious cats that Sandy loved so much.

I mentioned that we moved six times throughout my 36-year career and we picked up our four precious cats in four different cities. We met in Crescent City and we were married on February 5th. 1970 in Reno Nevada. Crescent City is on the coast in northern California. When you watch the news on television and the weatherman says it's raining near the Oregon border, that's where it's raining. Then we moved to Eureka and lived there from 1977 to 1986. Next we moved to Ukiah and we were there from 1986 until 1994. Ukiah is where we lived when Sandy brought home Sidney. Sidney is an all black male and he grew up to be a large cat (17 pounds). He is the most loving and also the most vicious of all our cats. Sidney ruled the household. He was king. Once when I went outside to bring Sidney back in the house, I reached down to pick him up and he wasn't ready to come in and clawed my hand. Needless to say, I let him stay outside a little longer while I went inside and washed the blood off my hand. Another time when I was at work, Sandy let Sidney go outside for a while and he got in a fight with a neighbor cat (he did that a lot). Sandy had to take him to the vet a few days later because he got an abscess in his neck. When I got home from work I sat down on the couch and Sidney came and sat on the floor in front of me. Sandy said, "Buddy, Sidney has something to show you." When I looked down at Sidney, I noticed that his neck was shaved and he had a tube sticking out of his neck. Of course I consoled Sidney about his wound and petted him. After I noticed and said, "you poor thing," Sidney went back to lie down on his favorite spot on the back of the couch. He didn't ask to go out (by standing in front of the door) until his wound healed., But as soon as Sandy took him back to the vet to have the tube removed, he wanted out again. Sidney is older now and doesn't go very far from home and he doesn't stay out very long. He still does and always has, liked to ride on my shoulder.

We then moved to Burney when I was promoted to store manager. We lived there from 1994 until 1997. Sandy came to me when we lived in Burney and said she wanted another cat. I said, "you had better get a female then, because I don't think Sidney would get along with another male cat." One day someone abandoned a calico kitten outside the place where Sandy worked and being the softy she was, she brought Isabella home. I think someone took her away from her mother too soon because she likes to nuzzle a lot and needs a lot of attention.

Next came Zoe, a black and white kitten. Sandy brought her home from the pound when we lived in Redding.

Sandy's employer and his wife went on vacation and put their dog in the kennel while they were gone. Sandy went to the kennel three times a week to pet their dog and bring it a treat. Sandy had to go by the cats to get to where the dog was kept and every day all the cats meowed at her except one. It just watched Sandy go by every day. On Sandy's last visit to the kennel, she stopped in front of the cat that didn't meow at her and said, "would you like to go home with me?" then the kitten meowed. So Sandy brought Zoe home. That was when we lived in Redding.

Zoe was just a small kitten and must have been very hungry, because she would fight Sidney for the food. Sidney just looked at her and let her eat. One time Sandy took a small piece of chicken from her plate at dinner time and reached down to give it to Zoe, Zoe bit Sandy's finger to the bone.

We were transferred from Redding to Rocklin and were there from 1999 until I retired in 2002. That's when we moved to our retirement home in Red Bluff. The first morning we woke up in our retirement home we saw thirteen deer and a flock of turkeys in our yard.

One night while I was checking my email I herd a noise outside the window in the garden area. I told Sandy about it and we went outside with a flashlight and found a little long haired black and white female kitten in our garden area. The kitten had burrs all over it so we brushed the kitten and fed it. It was so scared that it was still meowing when it ate. I fixed a place in the garage for it to sleep with some food and water and a litter box. The next day I put a sign up on the street that we had found a black and white kitten. Not to my surprise, noone claimed the kitten. Sandy asked me what I was going to do with the kitten and I told her that I would not take it to the pound because if noone claimed it they would put it to sleep. So we now had Sophie. Sophie loved Sandy and Sandy was the only one that could hold her. Sophie was scared of everyone else. Sophie finally warmed up to me and I could pet her but she still wouldn't let me hold her. When we had company Sophie would disappear to one of her favorite hiding spots and we would never see her until the company left.

Sandy loved her precious cats. Sandy had the three female cats declawed. She was tired of them tearing up the furniture. I put a piece of carpet on a board and screwed it to the wall for the cats to scratch their claws on but they still scratched on the furniture. I wouldn't let her have Sidney declawed though, he liked to roam sometimes when he was outside and I was afraid that he would meet up with another animal and be unable to protect himself or climb a tree. Sidney didn't sharpen his claws on the furniture anyway, he used the scratching post I built. Our cats were house cats but Sandy would let them play outside on nice days. She had them well trained, when she wanted the cats to come in the house she would just clap her hands and they would come running, except for Sidney. He wanted to stay out a little longer sometimes and we would let him because we could always get him in with the promise of food. As he got older, we didn't have to bribe him with food, he would always come in when we called him.

After we moved to Burney, Sandy and I would work in the yard on our days off. Of course we could only work in the yard on nice days in the summer time. Burney's altitude was 3200 feet and it snowed a lot in the winter.

Sidney was the only cat we had at the time and we would let him come outside with us as he would always stay close by. One day we worked outside all day long and when it came time to go in the house, we couldn't find Sidney. We searched the property, we had an acre, and couldn't find Sidney anywhere. We searched the surrounding neighborhood and Sidney was nowhere to be found. When it got dark, we had to come in the house. Sandy was hysterical. She was crying and was sure that Sidney was gone forever. I thought we would never see Sidney again but I didn't tell Sandy that. I was always optimistic about things and tried to comfort Sandy and assured her that Sidney was alright.

The next day I had to work but Sandy stayed home and searched for Sidney again. I called home several times to see if Sandy had any luck. There was no good news, Sandy still couldn't find Sidney. When I got home from work we searched again until dark and we couldn't find Sidney anywhere.

The third day went the same as the second, I had to work and Sandy stayed home to search for Sidney. When I got home from work, Sandy still hadn't found Sidney, so we searched until dark again. When we ended our search and started to go in the house through the back door, Sandy suddenly stopped and said that she herd Sidney meow. I didn't hear the meow and Sandy couldn't tell exactly where it was coming from so we turned around and walked toward the back fence when Sandy herd Sidney meow again. We were closer now and could tell where the sound was coming from. We looked up and there was Sidney thirty feet up a pine tree draped over a branch. The pine tree was just over our back fence on our neighbors property. Under the pine tree was our neighbor's three bear dogs and Sidney wasn't about to come down. We had a friend who worked for P. G. & E. And he was going to bring a company truck over with a lift and a bucket on it but his boss wouldn't let him. Sandy was hysterical and shaking, she grabbed the phone and called 411 and asked them what the number was for 911. They hung up on her. Sandy was kidded about that for a long time. I went and got my ladder and leaned it up against the tree, but it wasn't nearly long enough for me to reach Sidney. Sandy finally went to the neighbor and asked him to take his dogs out of the back yard so we could try and get Sidney out of the tree. He was very nice and put his dogs in the back of his pickup. We called and called Sidney but he still wouldn't come down. Then I had a brainstorm, I went into the house and got a can of cat food. I brought the can outside and said to Sidney, "yummy, yummy, yummy." Sidney knew what that ment and started to come down from the tree. He came down head first and after a few feet he fell. Like a dummy I put my arms out to try and catch him. Of course he fell with all claws fully extended and I ended up with a gash in my hand. Sidney ran into the house and we put out some food and water for him.

Sandy was still hysterical and called the Vet. And asked him what she should do. The Vet. Said to Sandy, "the cat will be fine as long as he drinks some water, but I suggest you have a drink."

5

The Rhino Head

When Sandy was home recuperating from her hospital stay, she didn't have the energy to resume her decorating genius. We talked about her most famous decorating success, "The Rhino Head."

When we lived in Redding, my friend Lance Butterman and I played in an Easter Seals charity golf tournament along with another coworker, Karen. The golf tournament was held at Twelve Bridges golf course, a three-hour drive for us so we had to get up early in the morning to make it on time. We arrived in time to warm up and visit with all our friends. They had putting contest, a long drive contest, and a closest to the pin contest. Lance won the putting contest and Karen won the long drive contest for women. Other than that we weren't good enough too win anything else. After the golf tournament there was a dinner and a raffle with a lot of really nice prizes that were donated for the raffle. There were golf clubs, golf bags, golf balls and a lot of other nice prizes to be won in the raffle including gift certificates to the pro shop. At the raffle one of the persons there won a plastic rhino head, we figured that it must have been a booby prize. Lance won two folding chairs to be used when waiting for his turn to hit the golf ball. Lance didn't figure he needed two chairs so he traded one of them for the plastic rhino head. We laughed so hard that we had tears in our eyes. After the raffle ended, we headed home and I think we talked and laughed about that rhino head most of the way home.

About a year after that I was transferred to Rocklin and my employees threw a going away party for me. They had the party at Lane and Clair's house and we had a barbeque and swam in his pool. There were a lot of my coworkers and friends at the party and it made me feel good. My coworkers took up a collection and bought me a going away gift, a gift certificate to the golf shop. They knew I loved to play golf and I loved the gift, because there was another golf club that I wanted. I made the customary speech about how nice it was to work with all of them and I meant it. Then lance brought out another gift from the employees. I opened it and what a shock it was. It was THE RHINO HEAD. We laughed and laughed about it. When my wife Sandy saw the rhino head she said, "I want that."

I reported to work in Rocklin on July 1' 1999. My company put me up in an apartment temporarily and Sandy stayed behind until our house in Redding sold. We listed it on Friday and I left for my new assignment on Sunday so I could get settled in and do some grocery shopping before I went to work on Monday. Sandy called me on Monday night at the apartment and told me that we had an offer on our house. She said that she made a counter offer and the potential buyers made another counter offer. Sandy said no the offer. She told our agent that she would not go any lower. Sandy thought I was mad at her for doing that but I really wasn't. I worked Tuesday and took Wednesday off so I drove home on Tuesday night after work. While Sandy and I were laying in bed talking about the last offer, the phone rang. It was our real estate agent, the people decided to take Sandy's last offer. We sold our home in three days, thanks to the good instincts of my wife. What good luck we had, but it had to be a tribute to Sandy's good decorating skills because the house was on the market for two years when we bought it. Selling the house so quickly made our transition to Rocklin easier, except now we had to find a place to live.

While the house was in escrow, Sandy made trips to Rocklin and stayed in the apartment with me. While I was working, Sandy looked at homes for us to buy. We had a time problem because the people who bought our house wanted a two-week escrow. So we (I mean Sandy) had to scramble and find a house quickly. We told our realtor our price range and he said that he didn't have any houses that cheap. Sandy looked on the internet and found several houses to look at and took the list to our realtor and asked him to show those houses to her. I didn't realize how much leg work went into looking for a new house until I retired and we moved to Red Bluff and I helped with the hose selection process.

Sandy found a house in Lincoln that she liked and had the realtor show it to me after work one day. I liked the house and we made an offer on it. Our realtor said that we should make a full price offer on the house because the homes there were selling fast. Our offer was accepted and we were able to move in at the same time the people moved into our house in Redding. The transition was smooth and we were able to get settled quickly. After we were settled, Sandy started her decorating genus.

The back yard was just a pile of dirt so we hired a contractor to put in a patio out there and another contractor to put up an arbor. Sandy designed the arbor and it was L shaped. All of our neighbors loved our arbor and some of them hired the same contractor to do one for them. Sandy planted some climbing plants at the posts, and they grew to cover part of the roof. We had to do this in two different years as we had to save our money for the next project. We also put a fountain in the back yard and it was peaceful listening to the fountain run when we went to bed. We put a table and chairs out there and had a lot of meals outside on nice days. That leaves us limited space in the backyard so Sandy did her gardening in pots. The next year we hired another contractor to put a sidewalk beside our house as it was just dirt too. We were on a corner lot and there was only 5 feet beside the house to the fence. Now it was all sidewalk. The other side was a bank and Sandy planted cypress trees just outside the fence and lavender on the bank.

On the inside, Sandy didn't like to see the kitchen from the dining room so I had to build a wall between the two. The dining room was originally a family room but we turned it into a dining room. The extra wall gave us more wall space in the kitchen so Sandy had her brother Sparky (the cabinet maker) build some kitchen cabinets to fill up the extra space the new wall provided. Sandy would spend hours at the paint store collecting samples of all the colors and bring them home and put them against the wall until she got just the right colors for the house. In our new dining room I built cabinets across one wall so Sandy could display her 13 sets of dishes and all of her stemware that she has collected over our 35 years of marriage. Then we ripped out all the carpets and I installed laminate flooring throughout the house and we used area rugs. I built cabinets in the garage to hold all my tools and still have room for the car. I just had to move the car out of the garage when I had some woodworking to do. Wood working has been my hobby for 25 years or so and I could have built the kitchen cabinets for her but she wanted her brother Sparky to do it. I have never seen any better work than that of Sandy's brother Sparky. Next came the guests' bathroom and Sandy decorated it in a jungle there and I had to mount the RHINO HEAD on the wall! It was beautiful. I think Sandy had that in mind when we acquired the rhino head.

After I retired and we had been in Lincoln for 3+ years, Sandy came to me and said, "Buddy, we have to move, this house is done and I don't have anything to do." So we put the house on the market and planned to move back to Redding where we have good friends. Property up north was also cheaper than where we lived so it turned out to be a good idea. So we put the house on the market and showed it several times. A single man looked at the house three or four times with the realtor and we were asked not to be there. The man (Jeff) even came by, introduced himself and told us how much he liked the house and the way it was decorated. He finally made a full price offer on our house and we accepted it.

There was, however, a condition. We had to leave the guest bathroom decorated the way it was and leave the rhino head! This was another stroke of genus by my wife Sandy.

We looked at houses in Redding but ended up buying a house in Red Bluff. The house we bought was a new construction and didn't have any landscaping, it was all natural. With the house being new I didn't think I would have to do any remodeling. Wrong, I first had to remodel all the closets, then move the washer and dryer to the garage, and build a wall between the kitchen and living room. Again, Sandy didn't want to see the kitchen from the living room. Then she trusted me to build the extra cabinet in the kitchen. By this time she trusted my work. Of course we had to paint all the walls a different color. Our efforts, however, were interrupted by Sandy's leukemia.

6

I Don't Want to Die

Finally July 23 Rolled around and we got up early that morning to make the three to four-hour trip to San Francisco. The clinic was across the street from the hospital and we arrived in plenty of time. We signed in and there was a black woman that helped us and she was the nicest person I think I've ever met, her name was Char. We came to look forward to seeing her every time we went to the clinic. We had to put our paper work in two different places. One was where they took Sandy's vital signs and the other where the nurses drew blood for testing. The nurses called us for the vital signs first and then for the blood tests. They suggested that we bring lunch to the clinic because we had to wait for the blood tests to come back before we saw the doctor.

The wait was only about an hour and during that hour the transplant coordinator came out to talk to us. Troy Nathan was the transplant coordinator. He was a registered nurse, wore glasses, stood about 5'8" tall, balding on top with brown hair around the sides. He had a medium build and was probably in his 40s, Or 50s. He sometimes wore a baseball cap and I asked him why. He said, "when I go outside my head gets cold, so I wear a baseball cap to keep it warm." Troy asked us about our insurance and when I told him what medical insurance we had he said, "don't worry, we negotiate a price with your insurance company and you'll never see a bill from us." I didn't worry about the money because Sandy's welfare was my main concern and the bills just didn't matter to me but I was glad that we were not going to get a bill from them.

We were shown to the Doctors' office and waited for him. We were seated at a round table with four soft chairs facing the doctor's desk. There were shelves on the wall to out right with some books and papers on them. The doctor's desk had a pile of papers on it and it looked a little cluttered. We met in his office because this was a family conference to determine what treatment if any Sandy was to receive and to discuss the potential risks and benefits of the stem cell transplant.

Doctor Chad Letterman came in to talk to us with the nurse coordinator Troy Nathan. Troy sat with us at the table while the doctor sat behind his desk. Doctor Letterman had grey hair, was probably in his fifties, slim to medium build and wore a stripped shirt and tie. Doctor Letterman was the head of the department and I felt good about that. Maybe it was the luck of the draw that we got the main doctor because there were seven or eight that rotated between the clinic and the hospital. Doctor Letterman talked about Sandy's leukemia at length and was very careful to fully explain everything. Sandy told the doctor that she wanted to be treated and cured, She said, "I don't want to die." Sandy also asked the doctor if she could be home by Christmas. Doctor Letterman told us that if the treatment went well that Sandy getting to go home by Christmas was a possibility. The treatment he recommended was an autologous stem cell transplant. The Doctor explained that an autologous stem cell transplant is an infusion of a patients own stem cells previously taken while the patient was in remission and stored (frozen). He went on to explain that they would infuse the stored stem cells back into Sandy after another round of chemotherapy. The infusion would be much like they would do a blood transfusion or give liquids intravenously.

Sandy still had a sense of humor after all she had been through because she told the doctor that all of her hair fell out with the last round of chemotherapy but she still had hair on her legs. Doctor Letterman said, "we'll take care of that." I asked the doctor if he was good at what he did and he looked a little shocked. I said, "that's a fair question" and the doctor said, "yes it is a fair question." He said, "yes, I'm good at what I do, we have had 197 leukemia patients and three have died, two were from infections and the other died of leukemia." I asked doctor Letterman what chance Sandy had of survival. Doctor Letterman gave her a 50-50 chance of surviving.

The blood tests came back and doctor Letterman said that Sandy was still in remission. The doctor wanted to start the treatment while the leukemia was in remission. In the mean time doctor Letterman wanted pre admission tests done to make sure that Sandy's body and organs were in good enough shape to withstand the treatment. Because of the distance involved, the doctor would allow some of the tests to be done at the hospital at home. Our favorite nurse practioner (Candy) said she would send for Sandy's medical records when she was in the hospital at home. She said that they may need the information later.

Some of the tests were:

- Blood tests: Complete blood count (CBC) and blood chemistries help measure different organ functions.

- Chest X-ray: an x-ray of the chest looks at the lungs, heart and surrounding structures for abnormalities.

- EKG: Electrocardiogram measures the heart's electrical impulses to evaluate rhythm and function.

- PFTs: Pulmonary function tests involve breathing in and out into different machines at different rates to evaluate lung function.

- Bone Marrow Biopsy: To make sure Sandy was still in remission.

The clinic made a return appointment for us on Aug. 9th. And they would get the rest of the tests at that time and probably admit Sandy to the hospital for her next round of chemotherapy on Aug. 12th., My birthday. We headed home with a very good feeling about the planned treatment. Sandy and I talked about it during the long drive home and were both excited about Sandy's treatment plan and chances of being cured.

During the next two weeks we had the required tests at the hospital in Redding and awaited out next doctor's appointment in San Francisco on Aug. 9th. We had the bone marrow biopsy in doctor Cambridge's office a week before our appointment in San Francisco.

During the nest six months I would make a total of 23 round trips to San Francisco. Some of the trips were with Sandy and when she was in the hospital I would make those trips alone. During those trips alone, I did a lot of thinking about Sandy's illness and our situation. I also remembered some of the good times we had with each other, our children, and our friends. Those good times are intermingled in the form of chapters in this book. Some of the good times I remembered are about me and my friends. I added those chapters because I wanted the reader to know what was going on in my mind during those months. Sometimes, on my trips, I would think about what Sandy was going through. During those times while I was alone, I could express my feelings without Sandy seeing how terrified I was. From time to time I would have to pull off the road to dry my eyes.

7

Matching Purses

I mentioned earlier that my friend Lance Butterman and I planned a trip to Las Vegas and we were worried if our wives would like each other. Lance and Eloise invited us to dinner because we enjoyed each others company and liked to get together once in a while. It also was a good time for the girls to meet and get to know each other. Eloise is a handsome woman, about my age (59), who retired from her government job about a year after I did. She was the budget director for either the city or county. I don't remember which. Her hearing was worse than mine and before she got hearing aids she couldn't hear a word I said unless she was looking at me. I thought it was just a blond thing. After she got her hearing aids, she couldn't believe how loud everything was, the birds, the wind, and the road noise when traveling in the car. She said that she liked her silent world and I agreed.

Lance and Eloise bought a house in the best neighborhood in town. He told me that he wanted to buy the worst house in the best neighborhood. They found one and it might have been the worst home but it was beautiful. The backyard was just dirt and they put a lot of money in it to make it more comfortable. They put a patio in with an arbor, a swimming pool with a waterfall, and landscaped the rest of the yard. Lance did the landscaping himself and it looked like a professional job.

Sandy and Eloise visited throughout the evening and found that they had one major thing in common. They both loved to shop.

While at dinner the girls overheard Lance and I talking about our planned trip to Las Vegas and Sandy said, "when were you going to tell us?" and Eloise said, "yea." We tried to get out of it by telling them we planned it as a surprise but I don't think they believed us. We talked it over and Sandy and Eloise thought the trip would be fun. Sandy and I had been to Las Vegas several times in the past and told Eloise what an exciting city it was. Sandy described some of the sights on the strip for Eloise and she became excited about going. They could go shopping while Lance and I went gambling. It looked like Sandy and Eloise hit it off and were going to like each other. So Sandy and Eloise saved their money for shopping and Lance and I saved up our money for trip expenses and gambling.

The big day came and we flew to Las Vegas together for a three night, four days stay. After our plane landed we took a cab to Paris hotel and casino and checked in. We went to our adjoining rooms and unpacked and cleaned up for dinner. We were going to stay in Paris that night and go visit other places the next day. When Lance and Eloise knocked on our door so we could go to dinner together, I answered the door. I had slacks, white shirt and a tie on. Lance had dockers and a polo shirt on and Eloise looked at Lance and Said, "I told you so." So Lance hung his head and went back to the room to change. We went downstairs to dinner and had a really nice meal. Sandy and I had stayed there before so we knew what to expect. Every hour or so the waiters and waitresses would go around the dinning room and sing. They would stop at some tables to sing to some of the dinners. We arranged it in advance for one of the handsome waiters to come and sing to Eloise. I think Sandy and I enjoyed it as much as she did. The girls stayed downstairs a little while and did just a little bit of gambling. They didn't want to do too much because they wanted to save their money for shopping. They went up to the room early because they were tired from the trip and Lance and I stayed downstairs and gambled. We stayed up until they kicked us off the table. We stayed because we both won some money and we went to bed happy.

The next morning we all met for breakfast, then the girls were off to go shopping. Sandy knew all the good places to shop and had a great time showing Eloise. Lance and I walked down one side of the street and back on the other visiting every casino and taking in the sights. Lance collected matchbooks so we picked one up at every stop. It was a long walk and we were worn out by the end of the day.

That afternoon we met Sandy and Eloise and recapped the events of the day. They each bought themselves a Louis Vuitton purse. The girls had matching purses. They told us about all the shops they visited and how much they enjoyed each others company.

Fine dining was one of our favorite things to do so we made reservations at Picasso's restaurant in "Bellagio's." All four of us agreed that it was the most wonderful dining experiences we ever had. We spared no expense and it was worth the several hundred dollars it cost us, especially since we won the money the night before. It was such a memorable and pleasurable experience that we all still talk about it to this day, and talk about doing it again someday. After dinner we saw Cirque du Soleil. It was a great day. It was a great vacation.

When we got home, I had a dream that we went back to Las Vegas with Lance and Eloise. When we got ready for dinner they knocked on our door and I had a suit on and Lance had a shirt and tie on. Eloise said, "I told you so." Lance hung his head and went back to their room to change. Then I dreamed that we went back again. When Lance and Eloise knocked on our door, Lance had a suit on and I had a tuxedo on. Eloise looked at Lance and said, "I told you so." So Lance hung his head and went back to their room to change. I told them about my dream and we had a good laugh about it.

8

Honeymooning

It was August 9. And we got up early again to make the trip to U.C.S.F.. We had a 1:00 appointment and when we checked in there were several receptionists. Sandy let someone else go ahead of us so we could talk to Char again. Char recognized us as she always did and said to Sandy, "how you doing baby, are you feeling OK?" On every one of our visits to the clinic we always looked forward to seeing Char. She is the nicest person I've ever met.

The clinic was on a hill in San Francisco, on the fifth floor, with windows all around the outside. What a wonderful view of the city we had. I could see the top of the Golden Gate Bridge and around the corner out another window I could see down town San Francisco and the Bay. Sandy still had two more tests that had to be taken, an EKG and a chest X-ray. We had to go to different floors for the tests and when we were done we went back to the fifth floor and waited for the nurses to take Sandy's vital signs and draw blood. Then we went back to the waiting room to wait for the blood tests to come back. Sandy took a banana or something to eat, but I didn't, so while we were waiting, I went down to the restaurant to get something to eat. When I got back up to the fifth floor, Sandy was still waiting to be shown to a room. After I found out how long the waits were going to be I started bringing a book to read.

The nurses finally took us to a room and we waited for doctor Letterman to come in. It seemed like a long time this time before he came to the room. Doctor Letterman finally came into the room and told us that he looked at Sandy's blood under a microscope and the Leukemia was back. Sandy looked at me when he said that and I was in shock, just looking down at the floor in total miss belief. I felt so helpless, it was just like the first time we found out Sandy had Leukemia all over again. I herd somewhere before that before you die your life flashes before your eyes. My life was flashing before my eyes and I wasn't the one at risk, Sandy was. But I was a part of Sandy and she was a part of me and if she didn't make it a part of me would die also.

I asked doctor Letterman, "how can that be, Sandy just had a bone marrow biopsy last week and it was clear?" Doctor Letterman said, "cancer cells grow very rapidly and they can come back fast." He also said that he would check with the other hospital about the medications Sandy received when she got her first round of Chemotherapy. Doctor Letterman called Leukemia cells "blasts". Immature white blood cells look like blasts so it's normal to have less than 5% blasts. Sandy has about 10% blasts so he was sure that the Leukemia was back. Doctor Letterman said, "I'm sending the blood tests to the lab but I'm sure they're going to agree with me." Doctor Letterman also said that each time the Leukemia comes back it's harder to treat.

Doctor Letterman said, "Your Leukemia is so aggressive that an autologous stem cell transplant wasn't the way to go, it wouldn't work." He said "we need to do an allogeneic stem cell transplant. I asked doctor Letterman, "does this change Sandy's odds of survival?" Doctor Letterman said, "yes, she has about a 30% chance of surviving the transplant, and another 30% chance of making it 100 days. After a patient survives for 5 years, we consider them cured.," "We just have to get Sandy in remission long enough to do the transplant." I asked doctor Letterman, "what if none of her brothers or sister is a match?" Doctor Letterman said "then we have to look for a non related donor."

An allogeneic stem cell transplant is where a stem cell donor is used to supply the stem cells. Troy Nathan, the transplant coordinator, came in to see us and ask if Sandy had any brothers or sisters. After Sandy gave him the information on her four brothers and sister, Troy said that he would send out kits to all of them to see if one of them would be a match. The kits would include all the supplies and instructions to send the six vials of blood each back to U.C.S.F. for testing.

The nurse practicioner said that they had to request Sandy's records a second time because the hospital at home didn't respond the first time. The records were received after the second request and she said that the hospital up north only used ½ the chemotherapy that they use at the University of California at San Francisco. I asked her if that meant that there was still hope and she said, "yes."

We waited for most of the day for a room in the hospital to become available because they were going to admit Sandy to the hospital for another round of chemotherapy.

Sandy always packed a bag with her five pairs of pajamas, underwear and slippers just in case she had to be readmitted to the hospital and she was going to be in the hospital this time for three to four weeks.

I spent the night in the hospital that night with Sandy, we laid in bed together and watched a movie. One of the nurses came in and saw us sharing the bed and went back out and told the other nurses that we were honeymooning. They knew she was kidding. The next day I drove back home and came back to visit Sandy in the hospital every four or five days. I would spent the night on each visit and do Sandy's laundry before I went back home. I was still sure that Sandy would come through this just fine.

I had mixed emotions about going back and forth between the hospital and home. When I was driving back and forth between the hospital and home is when I spent a lot of time thinking about our situation and about our past.

When I was at the hospital I wanted to be home, but I wanted to be home with Sandy. When I arrived home I wanted to be back at the hospital with Sandy. I loved her so much that I just didn't want to leave her.

Sandy was in the hospital for three weeks. After two weeks her body started to recover and make it's own red blood cells, white blood cells and platelets. When her blood counts were at an acceptable level, Sandy was released from the hospital and we went home for a month for her body to recover.

Sandy recovered very fast and seemed like her old self. On one of our weekly visits to the clinic, the transplant coordinator (Troy Nathan) said, "giving you Chemotherapy is like giving you water, you're handling the treatment well."

9

I Survived the Title Wave

I suppose at this stage of our lives and Sandy's treatment it is only natural to reflect on the past and think about the good times we had together, with our family and friends. While Sandy was in the hospital, I drove back and forth between home and the hospital. While driving I did a lot of thinking about the last 35 years of our lives together, much more than I've ever done before, I suppose it is because there is a chance I could loose her, but at this time I truly believe that she will be cured. I always seemed like I was in a daze, just staring at the road as I drove, but driving has always been good therapy for me. I don't remember any bad times, only the good ones, I suppose that's a good thing.

We did a lot of one time things with our children when they were growing up. All of the things we did with our kids are very fond memories for me and I'm certain that they are memorable for them as well.

In the 70s I was having a lot of trouble with my allergies and our family doctor made an appointment for me at an allergy clinic in Portland. We would have to stay there for a week and I would have to go through a series of tests to find out what I was allergic to. My appointments at the clinic were every morning for an hour. The doctor would do scratch tests on my back and then the next morning he would look at my back and determine how allergic I was to certain things. I don't remember how many things I was tested for but in the end I was allergic to dust, grass and animal hair. They prepared a serum for me and I would be taking allergy shots. After seven years of allergy shots my condition improved enough so that I wouldn't need to continue my allergy shots.

While we were in Portland, I only remember two things that we did with our kids, one of which was a fancy dinner at the top of the Hilton. We had lots of people waiting on us and the kids had a great time.

The second thing that I remember doing with the kids was taking them ice skating. It was the first time for all four of us and we fell down a lot. My son Michael skated around the rink at full speed, he had no fear. Sometimes his skates would flop over on their sides because it was hard to keep them upright. My wife, Sandy and my daughter, Nicole would skate around the rink holding onto the side rail. I just skated slowly and tried not to fall down. When the Zamboni machine came onto the ice all the skaters had to clear the ice. Sandy and Nicole were on the other side of the rink and it took them a long time to get off the ice and they were the last ones off.

Michael grew up to be a big hockey fan and goes to several San Jose Sharks games each year. Last year he took me to a game and I really enjoyed it. He was real disappointed this year when contract negotiations stalled and he had no hockey games to go to. Michael loves the sport and collects hockey memorabilia. He has a lot of stuff, hockey sticks, pucks, jerseys, and cards.

Once when we were on vacation we took our kids to Marriotts Great America. We took Sandy's youngest brother, Timmy, with us. Nicole was still pretty small then and we found a ride that I thought she would enjoy. She was just barely tall enough and when we put her on the ride she was all smiles. When the ride started she started screaming and continued throughout the entire ride. I almost had the attendant stop the ride so I could take her off.

There was one ride called the title wave and Sandy told the boys if they went on the ride she would buy them a t-shirt that said, "I survived the title wave" The ride was in a straight line with a big loop in the middle and the ends tilted upwards to stop the momentum and go back the other way. The ride went front-wards and then backwards and then they stopped the ride so that people could get off. The boys were afraid of the ride and at first they didn't want to go on it, but they wanted the t-shirt. Sandy wouldn't buy them the t-shirt unless they went on the ride so Sandy's brother Timmy wanted the shirt so bad that he decided he would go on the ride, but he wanted me to go with him. During the ride he clung to my arm the whole way, but he did it and Sandy bought him the t-shirt. Michael was real quiet after that. I knew he was thinking about going on the ride. Finally after an hour or so he decided that he wanted to go on the ride so he could get his t-shirt, but he wouldn't go alone so I had to go on the ride AGAIN. I didn't like it either time but I had to go on the ride twice so the boys could get their shirts.

We took our kids to Kirkwood once to go snow skiing. When we arrived we rented our skis went outside and waited for our lesson. We had an hour wait and the kids and I got tired of waiting and decided to go on the lift and ski back down the hill. When it was my turn to get on the lift, they had to stop it because I was in the wrong position. The attendant asked me if I had ever been on a ski lift before and I said, "no." She showed me how to get on and the lift proceeded up the hill. At the top of the hill I didn't have any trouble getting off but my daughter Nicole did. She just stayed on the chair and they had to stop the lift and back it up so she could get off. We then skied down the hill and it took us a while because we fell a lot. I learned how to snow plow and that helped me keep my balance. Snow plowing helped me a lot because I didn't go very fast but when I put my weight on my right foot, I turned left and when I put my weight on my left foot, I turned right. That was hard to get used to. We finally made it back to the bottom of the hill, just in time for the lesson. Sandy told me later that when she saw the lift stop, she thought that's my family and I said, "yes that was us." After the lesson the kids and I used the same lift and skied all day while Sandy skied down the bunny slope.

Another time when the kids were small, I read about the King Tut exhibit coming to San Francisco. I didn't know how to get tickets so I called my credit union, which was in the bay area and one of the ladies that worked there said she goes right by the place that sells tickets and she would pick some up for us. She was just wonderful and my wife sent her flowers at work. When we got the next newsletter we saw her picture in the newsletter with the flowers. The caption was "going above and beyond the call of duty." We appreciated it very much and she deserved all the credit and praise she received. We went to the bay area the night before we were going to see the exhibit and stayed in a motel. The next day we got up and ate breakfast, then drove to the exhibit. It was crowded and we had too follow the crowd, kind of like a herd of cattle. The kids were small so they could just squeeze in between the people and get up front for a good view. Nicole had to get up on her tiptoes to see but she seemed very interested.

One other time when we were on vacation we took our kids to a San Francisco Giants baseball game. It was a night game against the dodgers and we had tickets for the upper deck in right field. The wind was blowing pretty hard and when we got to our seats we were freezing. I don't think I've ever been colder. Now I knew why they sold those pins that said something about surviving a night game at Candlestick park. We were on vacation and we had the sleeping bags in the car, it's a good thing because I don't think we would have made it without them. So I had to go back to the car and get two sleeping bags. When I got back to the seats we bundled up in them. A little later I saw someone taking our picture, I think we must have made the news that night.

After Michael left home and joined the Air Force, I took Sandy and Nicole, our daughter, to another Giants baseball game. This time we went to a day game and sat in the lower section down the right field line. We were about ten rows from the front. That was when Vida Blue was playing for the Giants and between innings Vida Blue would come out of the bullpen and play catch with the right fielder. Nicole would go down to the railing and talk to him and she asked him for the ball. He said, "I can't give you the ball, honey." Nicole went down to the railing and talked to him between every inning. The security guard came and told her that she couldn't lean on the railing but she stayed there and talked to Vida Blue between innings. After Vide Blue was through playing catch with the right fielder just before the ninth inning, he looked up into the stands. I told Nicole, "stand up he's going to throw you the ball." Nicole stood up and Vida threw her the ball. After the game we went around back where the players came out and waited for Mr. Blue. Of course he was the last one out of the locker room. We approached him and Nicole asked him to autograph her baseball. He autographed the ball for Nicole and stayed and talked to us for quite some time. Vida Blue was very nice to us. It was a memorable day for all of us, especially for Nicole.

Sandy and I went on a cruise to the Bahamas after the kids grew up. I won the trip in a contest at the store. We flew to Miami and stayed the night in a hotel. We didn't leave the hotel that night we had dinner downstairs. I was so excited about the trip that I couldn't sleep that night. The next morning we had breakfast in the hotel and took a taxi to where we had to board the cruise ship. We were on the cruise for three nights and four days. We both had massages, played bingo, gambled a little and ate and ate and ate. We met another couple on the ship about our age and enjoyed their company. We had a vacation package that included a compact rental car and so did the couple we met. We combined our rental compact cars for one luxury car and drove to Disney world together. We had three days at Disney world and saw all the sights. We had lots of fun on the cruise but I think we both enjoyed Disney world more. It was a great vacation.

We also went to Hawaii for three weeks when Sandy's mother lived there. Sandy, the kids, and her mother wold go shopping or to the beach while I played golf on different golf courses. We did a lot of sight seeing and tourist stuff. We stayed on the main island the whole vacation and took in all the sights. Sandy's mother drove us all around the island. Sandy's mother took us to dinner one night to a restaurant that turned. It took an hour for the restaurant to make a complete circle. One day we went to a luau.

10

The Transplant

After Sandy's hospital stay in San Francisco, we spent a month at home so Sandy's body could recover before the next round of treatment. During that month we had weekly clinic appointments in San Francisco, and sometimes twice a week. During one of those visits the doctor gave us a three ring binder titled U.C.S.F. Bone Marrow Transplant Program. The chapters in the binder were: General information, directions to U.C.S.F., Members of the transplant team and how to reach them, understanding stem cell transplant, getting ready for the transplant, stem cell collection, Chemotherapy preparative regimen, your hospital stay, The transplant, Post transplant keeping healthy, infections, long term recovery, Medications, etc. All of the medical terms and explanations in this book came from the information in that binder.

We usually drove there and back on the same day but it was tireing so one time we stayed in a hotel room and went out for a nice dinner. At each appointment we looked forward to seeing Char, and she was always so nice to us. It was the same routine as before, they checked Sandy's vital signs and draw blood for testing. With each visit we would ask if the tests were done on Sandy's brothers and sister so we could know if there was a match. The blood samples came in one at a time and after the tests were run, Sandy had two matches. Her sister Dana and her brother William were both matches for Sandy. Sandy would say, "just call me lucky." Troy Nathan met us in the hall and had a calender or events for us and one for Dana. Dana would have Nuprigen shots for five days prior to stem cell collection. Nuprigen would help her body produce more cells and make them grow faster. Sandy would be admitted to the hospital on October, 10th. With the transplant to take place on October 19th. Dana was to start her Nuprigen shots on October 15th. And have the first four at home and the last one in San Francisco just before the stem cell collection. Troy said that he would send the Nuprigen and all the supplies to my home. He also said that there would be full instructions for the shots and I could probably give them to Dana or Dana could give them to herself. Dana felt more comfortable having the shots at the doctors office so she made the arrangements.

On our last visit to the clinic before Sandy was admitted into the hospital, doctor Letterman came in to tell us that the Leukemia was back. What a shock for both of us, I couldn't believe it and neither could Sandy. I felt just like I did the first time, what a letdown. I felt tired and drained, I felt helpless. Doctor Letterman said, "we have learned that we can not kill the Leukemia with chemotherapy". He went on to explain that we need to do full body radiation in addition to chemotherapy. Doctor Letterman made an appointment for us to talk to the radiologist before Sandy was to be admitted to the hospital that very day. Sandy was worried about having full body radiation and so was I, but it looked like our only chance. The radiologist explained that Sandy would only receive 1/6 the radiation that a lung cancer patient would receive. The radiologist went on to explain that they would take an x-ray of Sandy's chest and make lead blocks for the center of her lungs. Sandy felt a lot better after this meeting.

The radiologist went on to explain that total body irradiation is radiation given to the entire body in small radiation doses, two to three times a day, approximately four to six hours apart. A total of ten or eleven treatments depending on the rest of your treatment plan. Treatments are not painful and you will not feel anything unusual while the machine is on.

On October 10th. Sandy was admitted to the hospital. The groshong line had long since been removed so they had to put another line in (a triple line hickman catheter) it works the same way the groshong catheter did. The hickman catheter was put in by the surgical team the day after Sandy was admitted to the hospital. Sandy received nine doses of whole body radiation over five days. Then she received chemotherapy with high-dose etoposide given by vein over four hours. After a two day rest she received an intravenous infusion of stem cells from her donor, Dana. Sandy would receive two medicines aimed to prevent the development of graft vs. host disease against her body. Graft vs. host disease is where the donors stem cells would recognize Sandy's body as foreign and attack it. She would receive Tacrolimus (Prograf) intravenously during her entire hospitalization until she would be able to take pills by mouth. Tacrolimus is used to prevent rejection during liver transplants but is also used in stem cell transplants. Methotrexate would be given in four doses on days one, three, six and eleven after stem cell infusion. This time Sandy would be in the hospital for five to six weeks. I took the following information from the transplant binder the doctor gave us.

Direct side effects of chemotherapy and radiotherapy, from the information the doctor gave us:

• Chemotherapy with Etoposide causes a number of discomforts. Chemotherapy can cause nausea, vomiting and diarrhea. During the day of chemotherapy Sandy would receive anti-nausea medicines in an attempt to eliminate or reduce nausea and vomiting. These anti nausea medicines might make her drowsy.

• The high-dose therapy being used is expected to cause damage to hair, skin and the lining of Sandy's mouth and intestines. Hair loss was to be complete but temporary. In many cases the hair will grow back incompletely. During the first one to two weeks after bone marrow or stem cell transplantation there will be severe sores in her mouth. These the doctor explained would be painful enough to require morphine or other narcotics for pain control. Sandy would be completely unable to eat during this period of time and her nutrition would be maintained by intravenous feeding. The doctor said there will be irritation and sores throughout the entire intestinal tract which would also prevent Sandy from eating. This could also cause nausea, vomiting, diarrhea and crampy abdominal pain. Sandy could also develop a toxic skin rash affecting primarily the palms, soles and groin. The rash can be painful or blistering and Sandy may require morphine or other narcotics for pain control due to this rash. Her body will naturally heal from all of these high-dose chemotherapy related toxicities and this recovery would take approximately one to three weeks.

• High dose chemotherapy and radiation can cause damage to internal organs as a direct toxicity of this treatment and if this damage occurs, it could be disabling or even fatal.

Complications of low blood counts:

• Much of the danger associated with high-dose chemotherapy or radiation treatments are the complications of lowered blood counts. The high-dose treatment Sandy was to receive would completely stop her own bone marrow from producing blood cells. It would actually kill all of her bone marrow. There was to be a period of approximately two to four weeks before her new infused bone marrow starts to grow and function effectively. Low white blood counts leads to vulnerability in infections since white blood cells protect against infection. Sandy would be receiving antibiotics to try to prevent and treat those infections. However, occasionally an infection could become overwhelming and even fatal. Sandy would require transfusions of red blood cells because of anemia. Sandy would also require transfusions of platelets to prevent bruising and bleeding. There is a danger where her body might not accept platelet transfusions from other people, and there may be a risk of serious or even fatal bleeding.

Failure to engraft:

- The high-dose chemotherapy/radiotherapy treatment Sandy was to receive would permanently damage her own bone marrow so that it would never grow back. Restoration of her bone marrow function and blood counts will require the re-growth of the infused bone marrow from her sister Dana. If this bone marrow fails to grow properly she could suffer from bone marrow failure (anemia, low white blood count and platelet count) which could be disabling or possibly fatal. That risk however was less that 1%.

Troy Nathan told us that we would have to spend two to three months in an apartment in San Francisco after the transplant. In case something goes wrong we have to be close to the hospital. Troy set up an appointment for us with the councilor. The councilor asked us a lot of personal questions and I told her about driving back and forth. She then asked Sandy if she was ok with those arraignments. Sandy said that she was. I suppose the councilor was trying to assist us but we both wondered why we had to meet with a councilor. The councilor gave us information on temporary housing and we called around and secured a furnished apartment for us to live in.

Sandy is the most courageous person I know, she never once complained and did everything the doctors told her to do. Sandy had a very strong desire to live and I knew that would be a factor in her favor during her struggle with Leukemia. The doctors gave Sandy a 30+% chance of survival.

After Sandy was admitted to the hospital I stayed two nights and three days each week when I visited her. I did her laundry when I visited her and we would talk about the events that took place when I went home. She would always ask me how the cats were doing and they would always be fine. I just hated to be away from her and after a while I would stay longer on each visit. I would only go home for long enough to check on the house and cats and pay bills.

I had made motel reservation for Dana for the day before the stem cell collection was to take place. I drove her to San Francisco and checked her into the motel. Dana's boyfriend was going to meet her there that afternoon and deliver her the next morning, so after checking Dana into the motel I drove to the hospital and spent the night with Sandy.

Information from the transplant binder.

Blood Stem Cell Harvest:

A process called apheresis is used for blood stem cell harvest. The term "apheresis" means blood cell separation. An apheresis machine will collect some of Dana's white blood cells. The blood cell harvest is performed in an outpatient setting. In this process, blood is continuously removed through one lumen of her catheter separated by the apheresis machine, and returning through the other lumen of her catheter. Stem cells are collected in a special holding bag. The stem cells are then given immediately.

About 9 ½ ounces of blood was outside her body during the procedure. This collection of WBCs will include stem cells. Only one collection would be taken per day and she would be connected to the machine for 3-5 hours.

To prevent her blood from clotting when it is moving through the apheresis machine a citrate solution would be added. Citrate binds some of her body's calcium and could cause tingling in her lips, fingers, or toes. Dana was instructed that if any of these symptoms were to occur she was to let the nurse know and the nurse would provide additional calcium. It was explained that these symptoms are generally mild and would resolve quickly. To help avoid these symptoms she was instructed to eat extra dairy products during the week before the apheresis. Dana's blood would cool down slightly while it is circulating through the machine and she could feel chilled as the blood is returned to her. Dana was instructed to dress in layers as that may allow her to adjust to temperature changes.

Once she was "hooked up" to the machine she could not be disconnected until the collection was complete. She was advised to use the restroom before the procedure and avoid diuretics such as coffee, tea, and sodas before the procedure.

Dana was to meet the transplant coordinator the next morning at 7:00 A.M. Dana was to have a Central Venous Catheter like Sandy's put in so the doctors could remove the stem cells needed for the transplant. Then Dana was to be back at the hospital at 2:00 that afternoon to begin the stem cell collection. On the way back from having the Central Venous Catheter surgically put in Dana noticed that she was bleeding so she went to the clinic to have them look at it. They fiddled around with it for a while and thought they had the bleeding stopped. The stem cell collection took place as scheduled and she was free for the rest of the day. Dana was to return at 7:00 A.M. the next morning for another round of stem cell collection. The doctor wanted to make sure that he had enough and they would freeze some in case they were needed at a later date. That evening Dana and her boyfriend (Bart) went to the motel to get ready to go out to dinner. Bart is an electrician and is in his late 40s. Or early 50s. Dana noticed that she was still bleeding so they went to the emergency room at the hospital.

That night I call the motel to check on Dana and see how she was doing and there was no answer. Sandy became worried and told me to find her and see if something was wrong. I called the emergency room to see if she was there and she was. I went down to the emergency room to see what was wrong. When I got there she was still waiting for the doctor and she was still bleeding. The emergency room had to call the head of cardio-vascular surgery in to fix the problem. Evidently the surgeon that put the catheter in nicked a vein and that was what caused the bleeding. When the head of cardio-vascular surgery got there, Dana was skeptical and said to him, "I hope you don't mind me asking but do you know what you're doing?" the Doctor said, "don't worry this is my specialty." The specialist had to put a stitch in to keep it from bleeding. When I found Dana I had to go back up to her room and give her a report. Then I went back down to the emergency room to check on Dana's progress. When it looked like everything was going to be taken care of I went back to the room and told Sandy everything was alright.

I was sleeping in Sandy's room that night in a chair that folded flat when I woke up in the middle of the night to go to the bathroom. I herd snoring and it sounded like Sandy, but Sandy was sitting straight up in her bed. I thought, how could Sandy be snoring if she is awake? They had put Dana in Sandy's room also and she was the one snoring. It sounded just like Sandy. Sandy was watching Dana to make sure she would be alright, I think she stayed awake all night. That was Sandy for you, always worrying about other people and not herself.

The next morning the nurse came to get Dana so they could do another stem cell collection. When I woke up she was gone and Sandy wanted me to go check on her. The collection was to be held on the ninth floor and we were on the eleventh floor so I went two floors down to check on Dana. I talked to her and she hadn't eaten in 24 hours so I went down to the cafeteria and got her some breakfast and brought it up to her. After the second round of stem cell collection, the doctors took out the Catheter and she was released to go home. That was quite an experience for Dana but she said that she would do it again for anyone and I said, "so would I."

The transplant took place at 2:00 that afternoon and was anticlimactical. I then went home to take care of the house and the cats.

The nurses drew blood everyday to check Sandy's blood counts and give her transfusions if needed until her body started producing blood again. Or I guess it would be Dana's cells taking over and producing red and white blood cells and platelets. Sandy would have Dana's immune system now.

More information from the binder:
Waiting for Engraftment:

It would take approximately two to three weeks for Sandy's (Dana's) bone marrow to start producing white blood cells, red blood cells and platelets.

Engraftment is the term used to describe when the patients new marrow begins to function and produce cells. During this time, no mature cells leave the marrow and enter the blood stream. Sandy's blood counts would show very low values and she would require careful monitoring by the healthcare team. The goal is to support her with red blood cells and platelets until her body begins to produce cells again.

When her red blood cell count is too low, she will receive packaged red blood cell transfusions. These consist of a bag or bags on concentrated red blood cells; each bag transfused over 2-3 hours. This means that Sandy and the donor have the same type of blood. All blood products are carefully tested for all types of hepatitis, AIDS, (human immunodeficiency virus or HIV) and syphilis according to the federal requirements. Cytomegalovirus (CMV) testing would also be done if her doctor decided it is needed.

When Sandy's platelet count is low, she will receive platelet transfusions. These consist of a bag or bags of platelets infused over approximately 15 minutes.

Sandy could sometimes experience and uncomfortable reaction to her blood product transfusions. Some of these reactions are fever, chills, and shaking, itching, and skin rashes. Infrequent side affects are back pain and shortness of breath. The red blood cells and platelets are irradiated and filtered and frequently medications may be used before the transfusion to minimize any side affects. Sandy would be monitored carefully for any of these reactions.

11

The Doubleheader

On my drives back and forth from home to San Francisco, I thought about Sandy all the time. I never did think that she would die, I always thought she would be cured. I had a lot of time to think about our life together and how much I loved her. I thought about a lot of things, this one involved my friend lane and myself.

Sandy and I hadn't been married long when she found out how much I like sports. I was a 49er. Football fan and on Sunday's I would be glued to the T.V. Sandy would be waiting for us to do something together on my day off and finally realized that I wasn't going to budge from the T.V. so being the wonderful wife and person she was, she finally sat down beside me and started asking me questions. Her questions were mostly about the penalties and what they meant. Sandy, over time, became as big a fan as I was. When the 49ers. Beat Dallas in a championship game that featured "the catch", Sandy went around the neighborhood with champagne for all the neighbors. The catch was a touchdown pass thrown by Joe Montana to Dwight Clark to win the game.

Once when we lived in Redding, I had to go to Sacramento on business. I drove down to Sacramento the night before and Sandy went with me. As we were driving by Arco Arena, I noticed that the lights were on. I asked Sandy, "do you want me to call when we get to the hotel and see if there is a game tonight?" Sandy said, "OK." When we got to the hotel we unpacked and settled in and then I called the arena to see if there was a game and if there were tickets available. I found out that there was a game and that there were ticket available, so after dinner we drove to the arena paid for parking and walked to the ticket window. When I got up to the ticket window I asked the clerk what seats were available and he showed me several seats to choose from. I don't know what made do it but I then asked him if he had any front row seats available. The clerk showed me a seating chart of the arena and gave me a choice between two different sets of seats. I said, "I'll take these two" The clerk then printed up the tickets and said to me "that will be $410 for the pair. I didn't realize that front row seats to a basketball game cost so much so I just stood there for a moment. Finally I thought what the heck and pulled out my wallet and slid my credit card under the window. Tickets are a lot more than that now and I don't think I'll be doing that again. We watched the Sacramento Kings game from the front row and it was a terrific experience, we both loved it. We didn't even have to get up to go buy drinks or snacks, we had a waitress that came around and took our orders. Sandy was enjoying the game so much that at halftime she told me to go upstairs and buy some more tickets for a future game. So I went upstairs and bought two more front row tickets for a Laker game a month or so in advance. We still talk about that experience with our friends to this day.

When we moved from Redding to Lincoln, I met and became friends with two retired football players. Cedrick Hardman and Jerry Robinson came to the store for a weekend to sign autographs for charity. Cedrick Hardman was a defensive end for the San Francisco 49ers. And Oakland Raiders and Jerry Robinson was a linebacker for the Philadelphia Eagles and the Oakland Raiders I think that Cedrick is still the quarterback sack leader for the 49ers.

Cedrick Hardman gave me two tickets to a 49ers. Game. It was a Sunday night game against the New Orleans Saints. Sandy didn't want to go to the game. After 9-11 she wouldn't fly or go anywhere there were a lot of people. I asked my friend Lane Yeperson to go with me and he was very excited to be able to go. Lane lived in Redding and came down to spend the night before the game with me. We had dinner and Lane said," Buddy, let's get up early and go by Pac Bell Park." I said, "sounds like a good idea to me." So we got up early, ate breakfast and went on our way to the ball park.

The San Francisco Giants were playing their last game of the season and it was against the Dodgers. We got to Pac Bell park in plenty of time for the game and bought tickets. Of course our tickets were in the nose bleed section but that was ok. We bought our nacho's and beer and went to our seats just in time to see Barry Bonds hit home run #73 for the season. We spent the rest of the game walking around the ball park watching the game from different viewpoints. We walked out to the outfield but the security guards had it roped off. They wouldn't even let people walk through unless they had a ticket. We watched Barry Bonds take his turn at bat in the eighth inning and then left for Candlestick Park to watch the 49ers. Play.

The 49er. Saint game started at 5:00 P.M. because it was on television. We got to the park real early and found our seats and waited for the game to start. It was a great game, probably because the 49ers. Beat the Saints. When there was three minutes left in the game I said to Lane," let's go, you have to work tomorrow and if we wait until the game is over it'll take us two hours to get out of the parking lot." Lane was hesitant because he wanted to watch the rest of the game but he finally gave in and we left. We got to the car just in time to hear the end of the game and we had no trouble getting out of the parking lot and onto the freeway. I'm sure that leaving early saved us at least two hours. We talked about our doubleheader all the way home and still do to this day.

WHAT A DAY!

12

The Apartment

About two weeks after Sandy had her transplant our doctor came in to see Sandy and told her that we had graft. That was good news, Sandy was all smiles and she was excited. I was just as excited as she was. All we had to do now was to wait for Sandy's new stem cells to start making new red, white blood cells and platelets. I kept in close touch with the doctors because I had to call and rent the apartment. I had already paid my deposit but had to tell them when I would be moving in as soon as I had a date. We had to be close to the hospital after the transplant because the doctor told us that it was not uncommon for a patient to have to go back to the hospital at least once and we had to be within an hour of the hospital in case of an emergency.

Sandy's blood counts were coming up nicely and doctor Letterman gave us a release date of Nov. 7th. I called and rented the apartment for three months beginning November 5th. I went home one last time to take care of the cats and pay the bills. Dana was going to take care of our cats and pile the mail up on the kitchen table for us. Sandy had packed a suitcase for herself on our last trip home together so I packed one for myself and loaded the car for the trip to San Francisco. I drove down on November 5th. And I met the agent. He took me to the apartment and showed me around. After he gave me the keys, I unloaded the car and unpacked our suitcases. I then drove to the hospital to be with my wife.

The pharmacist came in and covered the prescriptions that were called in to the pharmacy and explained what they were for and the side effects. The medications that were prescribed were:

* Tacrolimus .5mg. Twice a day, this medication may cause diarrhea, insomnia or headaches. Tacrolimus may increase blood pressure and cause tremors, long term therapy may increase chances of diabetes. This medication will decrease your body's chances of fighting infections, so try to avoid those who are sick and large crowds. Do not drink cranberry juice or grapefruit juice while taking this medication.

- Voriconazole 250 mg. Twice a day to treat fungal infection. Call your doctor in you experience any decrease in vision or blurred vision. This medication may cause nausea or upset stomach, may cause headache.

- Dapsone 100mg. Tablets. An antibiotic.

This medication may cause nausea or vomiting. This medication may cause numbness in the extremities. Space medication from antacids at least two hours apart.

- Atenolol 25mg. Tablets for high blood pressure.

- Magnesium oxide 400mg. Tablets. Two tablets twice a day. Tacrolimus uses up the magnesium in your body, this replaces it.

- Rabeprazole 20mg. Tablets for stomach protection or reflux.

- Prochlorperazine 10mg. Tablets as needed for nausea.

- Potassium Chloride.

- Lorazepam 1mg. Tablet as needed for mild nausea.

- Acyclovir 200mg. Tablets three times a day an anti-viral medication.

I just listed the medications to show how many pills Sandy had to take each day. Sandy has never been a pill person, they always upset her stomach so I knew she would have trouble. The pharmacist told us that it was important to take all the medication exactly as described. We were to call the clinic if Sandy missed or was unable to take even a single dose. Sandy wanted to be in charge or her medications and didn't want me to get them ready for her.

After visiting with Sandy in the hospital and meeting with the pharmacist, I spent the night in the hospital. The next morning I went to the pharmacy to pick up the prescriptions and then to go grocery shopping. I wanted to take care of all the errands before Sandy was released from the hospital so I wouldn't have to leave her once she was released.

I picked Sandy up from the hospital on November 7th. As scheduled and we went to live in the apartment. I told her that I would not leave her side for at least three weeks as Dana was taking care of the cats and the house. I don't know what we would have done if it hadn't been for Dana taking care of the cats and mail for me. She was a lifesaver, in more ways than one. The only time I wasn't with her was when I had to go to the grocery store or run some errands and then for an hour or less. I loved her so much that I just wanted to take care of her. On one of my errands I bought a D.V.D. player so we could watch a couple of movies that I bought while I was at the grocery store. I told our daughter Nicole that she could have it when we left the apartment as we had one at home.

I would buy Sandy anything she wanted and I would cook anything she wanted to eat even though I had never cooked before. She told me that I got pretty good at it. Sandy was my whole life and I wanted to make her happy. I cared for her in every way that I could. There was only one good thing that came out of Sandy's illness: it brought us closer together than we had ever been before.

Sandy had trouble taking all of those prescriptions, they made her stomach upset. One day she told me that she didn't think that she could take them anymore. I told her tat if she couldn't take the pills, she would have to go back into the hospital so they could give her the medication intravenously. She never complained after that, she just took her pills the best she could because she didn't want to go back into the hospital.

There was a courtyard behind our apartment with a cement walkway in a circular shape with grass in the middle. The weather in San Francisco was surprisingly warm for that time of year and the weather never kept us from going for a walk. There was a golf course behind the apartment, I think it was the Olympic Club. Golf was the last thing on my mind so I didn't even try to play. I didn't even think about golf while Sandy was sick. Sandy would push herself to do twelve laps a day, but she wasn't as healthy as she had been after the first two rounds of chemotherapy, it was taking it's toll on her body. She knew how much I loved her, I told her every day, and I knew how much she loved me. It's hard to describe what I'm feeling right now, I love her so much. It was not just my duty to take care of her, it was my pleasure. Sandy was worried about me having to take care of her and I told her," you took care of me for thirty five years, I can take care of you for one." That seemed to put her mind at ease.

After Sandy was release from the hospital we had clinic appointments twice a week. We went to the clinic on Tuesdays and Fridays and we always looked forward to seeing our favorite receptionist, Char. The routine was always the same, we would check in, the nurses would take Sandy's vital signs, draw blood for testing and then we would wait to see the nurse practioner. While we were waiting I would go get the paper to read and a Starbucks coffee or go to lunch. We would always ask for our favorite nurse practioner Sherry. Sherry would check the results of the blood tests and adjust Sandy's medication as needed. Sandy's magnesium would always be low so she would infuse magnesium intravenously. The pills weren't enough so Sherry ordered supplies for us so I could infuse magnesium at the apartment in between clinic appointments. The nurses trained me how to infuse the magnesium. Sandy still had her triple line hickman so I had to flush the lines daily with heparin. I would have to wash my hands with antibacterial soap for fifteen seconds and then use an alcohol swab to clean the end of the line with before I flushed it or infused the medication. I would have to flush the line I was going to infuse the magnesium with a saline solution before and after the magnesium and then flush with heparin.

Sandy was doing pretty good and every trip to the clinic showed no signs of Leukemia. So after three weeks I planned to go home for 24 hours and pay the bills and check on the house. I couldn't leave Sandy alone and the doctor said it was too soon to take her that far away from the hospital so I asked my friends Lance and Eloise Butterman to come to the apartment and stay with Sandy while I went home. I planned the trip between clinic trips so Lance and Eloise wouldn't have to take Sandy to a clinic appointment. I did her infusion of magnesium before I left and would do the next day's when I got back. I put dinner in the crock pot for them that morning and when they got there I took off for home. Sandy taught Lance and Eloise how to play cribbage while I was gone. I hated to be away from Sandy but I had to go through the mail and pay the bills. When I got home the kitchen table was piled high with newspapers and mail. I didn't have time to read the papers so I put them in the recycling bin. I stayed up until 2:00 A.M. to get through all the mail and pay the bills. I got up early the next morning and drove back to San Francisco. When I got back to the apartment Lance and Eloise had dinner planned for us. Lance and I went to the store to by some Dungeness crab while Eloise stayed with Sandy. They had dinner with us and stayed the night. The next day they went shopping in San Francisco before they went home.

At our next clinic appointment I asked doctor Letterman if I could sneak sandy home for a 24 hour visit. Doctor Letterman said, "it should be ok in a couple of weeks." So, I planned my next trip home in two weeks and Sandy would go with me. I was excited about Sandy getting to go home for a day because I knew she wanted it.

After the two weeks past we went home for the day I took Sandy's I.V. stuff so I could infuse her magnesium while we were at home. Sandy was so glad to be home and to be able to sleep in her own bed. And she was so excited to see her precious cats and they were happy to see her. Just like the last time, Sandy didn't have an empty lap the whole time with Sophie taking up most of the time while Sandy crochet on her baby blanket. Sandy didn't have anyone special to give the baby blankets too, she just crochet them and put them away. She did give a lot of them away as friends had baby's.

We were Sacramento Kings fans and once she read that Doug Christie's wife was pregnant she took one of her baby blankets to a game with her and gave it to a security guard and asked him to give it to Doug Christie. Doug Christie was a Sacramento Kings basketball player. Sandy was always doing nice things for other people, even people she didn't know.

When we went home for our 24 hour visit, Sandy got out all of her jewelry and some of her personal items and divided them up and put names on them. She also wrote me a 5 page note that described who she wanted all of her personal stuff to go to in case something went wrong and she died. I told her that she wasn't going to die, but I would follow her wishes to the letter. So I put the note in my desk. The next morning we were off to go back to the apartment in San Francisco.

Doctor Letterman originally gave Sandy a 30% chance of making it through the transplant, and another 30% chance of making it 100 days, and another 30% chance of making it a year. After 5 years they would consider Sandy cured. I asked doctor Letterman on one or our clinic visits, "does this mean that Sandy has made it through the first phase?" Doctor Letterman said, "I would say yes." That was good news for both of us and made us feel a lot better.

Nicole was coming over to the apartment for thanksgiving dinner and we were going to have turkey, stuffing, mashed potatoes and asparagus. Sandy was feeling good that day and at dinner she went back for seconds. Nicole and I looked at each other in amazement, we both couldn't believe that Sandy was eating so much. It was a good day.

13

The Award

In the apartment, we reminisced a lot about the past. One of the things we talked about was Sandy's most important accomplishment, her major award.

When the kids were almost grown, Sandy said that she didn't want to be at home alone so she went out and got a job. We lived in Ukiah at the time and Sandy applied for a job at J. C. Penney's. She went for an interview and they hired her. She came home that night and told me that she got the job and hoped that they didn't put her in shoes. She said that she would enjoy working in any other department, just not shoes. She went to work the following Monday and they put her in shoes. Sandy is a good employee and she worked hard and became a merchandisers assistant.

Each year for the month of October, Sandy's company would have a contest for all the merchandising assistants, so Sandy put together a merchandising plan for the month. She developed large displays, centered around a new shoe style each week. The first week she featured men's and ladies dress shoes. The second week she featured western boots. The third week she featured athletic shoes and for the final week she developed a massive displays of shoes.

For the contest Sandy established competitions for individual sales, credit applications, and catalog referrals and book sales. She also coordinated weekly merchandise statements with upcoming ads to generate selling activity. For the month her department posted a 51% sales gain. Sandy's manager said, "concern for customers, that's the key to Sandy's success, she takes care of them immediately. Customers sense her concern and, consequently, love to shop in her department."

Sandy won the store contest and the store manager brought her flowers and told her that her entry and results would be entered into the district wide contest. Sandy's manager informed her a week later that she had won the district wide contest and that her plan and results would then be entered into the regional wide contest. For winning the district wide contest, Sandy received a plaque and

$100. She then won the regional wide contest and received an inscribed crystal vase and $200. Then her entry was entered into the company wide contest. SHE WON! Sandy received $200 and an engraved silver bowl. They also flew us to Las Angeles for a trip to Disneyland. The night before we went to Disneyland we were invited to have a dinner reception with the company's top executives including the C. E. O. There were several tables set up and one top executive sat at each table. The company's top human resources manager sat at our table. Sandy was very good at what she did and I was so proud of her. She won the company's top award.

When Sandy went back to work the following Monday, her department manager (William) was waiting for her and eager to hear all about our weekend. Sandy told William all about our weekend and told me later that William was green with envy. William wanted to know if we met the C.E.O. and Sandy said, "yes." William had never met the C.E.O. of the company and wanted to know what he was like. Sandy told William that we talked to him for about ten minutes and that I was going back down south to play golf with him the next weekend. Sandy was teasing William and he thought that I was going to play golf with the C.E.O. on a regular basis. Sandy never told William that she was teasing him.

Sandy went on to manage a privately owned shoe store and once she brought home the diagrams of the bones in a foot. I was watching something on T. V. And noticed Sandy studying something so I went over to see what she was doing and she was studying the diagram. Sandy gave her all to whatever she did and studying that diagram confirmed that.

One of the Podiatrists in town would send his patients into the shoe store, that Sandy managed, for a certain shoe. Sandy looked at the shoe the doctor wanted his patient to have and thought she had a shoe better suited for her. Sandy gave the lady the shoe and asked her to show it to her doctor. The doctor called Sandy the next day and told her that he wanted all of his patients to have the shoe that Sandy recommended.

Once we were at a wine tasting and a concert in the grass sitting on a blanket drinking wine and listening to the music, when the man in front of us got up and walked away. I think he was going for more wine or something. Sandy noticed the way he walked and leaned forward to talk to his wife. Sandy said that by the way he walked she could tell something was wrong. She asked the lady if his feet were bothering him. I didn't listen in on the conversation, I could only hear Sandy's side of it. Sandy told the lady that her husband should come in and see her because she had a pair of shoes that would work for him. Sandy suggested that he might see a doctor because she said that sooner or later his knees would start bothering him and then later his hip would start bothering him. I don't know whether they came in to see Sandy or not. Sandy didn't just go to work she studied her profession and knew it well. There was no doubt in my mind that Sandy was right because she was so good at what she did.

She told me about the time a man and a woman came into the shoe store to buy a pair of shoes for the man. He was rather rude and Sandy said that he didn't want to be there, but he reluctantly tried on several pairs of shoes. Sandy told me that he said he wore a size 8 ½ and wouldn't let Sandy measure his foot. She said that she could tell by looking that he wore a bigger size than 8 and ½. Sandy told me that they were there for over an hour, and finally she brought out shoes that she thought would be good for him instead of the ones he wanted to look at. Without saying anything to the man she brought out a bigger size of shoe (I think a 9 or 9 ½) and the man couldn't believe how good they felt. The grumpy old man left happy and said that he wouldn't go anywhere else but there for shoes. Sandy wasn't only good at what she did, she was excellent at customer service as well.

14

The Goof Troop

As I said earlier, I thought about a lot of things during my 3-4 hour drives back and forth from the hospital and home. Sometimes I not only thought about Sandy, but I thought about my life and what it would be like without her. The goof troop is another one of those memories I relived in my mind. I'm attempting to share not only how I acted, handled, and coped with the tragic situation, but also what I was thinking.

I had always played golf with Lance and once in a while with Lane. When I retired and moved to Red Bluff Lance and I played golf once a week, weather permitting. Lance had two friends, Jack Smith and Bart Cummings. Jack is a retired police officer from the Los Angeles area. Jack is a little taller than I am and a little heavier but not much. Bart is about the same height as I am but a little thinner. I don't know where Bart retired from but we are all retired. We all have a little grey in our hair but Bart's hair was white. We all get together once a week weather permitting to play golf, usually on a Tuesday. Tuesday was a discount day at the golf course and we get a good rate to play. Bart likes to travel a lot so sometimes there are only three of us. We like each others company and joke around a lot. We have fun on the golf course and always complement each other on good shots. Jack is the best golfer of the four of us and the rest of us are about equal. Sandy hadn't met Jack or Bart at this time so I told her about them and our antics on the golf course, so she called us the goof troop. She even planned to make the four of us t-shirts that said goof troop on them.

When Eloise retired there was a retirement party for her. It was a luncheon and a lot of the city officials were there. Jack and Bart were also there and I took Sandy over to meet them. Lance was talking to them at the time so all four of us were together when I introduced Sandy. Sandy said, "so this is the goof troop, what a combination of characters." We all had a good laugh.

After Sandy was diagnosed with Leukemia, Jack went for his yearly physical and the doctor told him that he thought he had prostate cancer. It was confirmed by a specialist and he later had it removed. His recovery period seemed like a long one and after he began to feel better, Jack and Lance came to my house to putt on my putting green and have lunch with me. Sandy was home for recuperation after her first hospital stay and had lunch with us. Sandy and Jack talked a lot about their fights with cancer.

15

The Most Courageous Person I Know

On December 14th. We got up and went to one of our twice a week clinic appointments. We arrived at the clinic just after 9:00 A.M. and as usual Sandy had her vital signs taken and her blood drawn for testing. Then we waited. Her magnesium was low so the nurse came and showed us to a room. The nurse gave her some magnesium intravenously over two hours. After the infusion was finished we waited what seemed like a very long time before the nurse practioner came in to see us. She said that the doctor wanted to see us and I thought that could only be bad news. I stopped another one of the nurse practioners in the hall and told her that the doctor wanted to see us and I asked her if it was going to be bad news again. She said to me, "is it always bad news when the doctor see's Sandy?" I said, "no, not always." She didn't know what the reason was that the doctor wanted to see us. We waited and waited.

Finally the doctor came to see us and he told us that the Leukemia was back again. I couldn't believe it. Good news then bad news then good new and then bad news again. Each time was worse than the first. I asked the doctor if we had any treatment options left and he said, "yes, we only had one." I asked the doctor if it was time to give up and he said, "no, I'll tell you when it's time to give up." Doctor Letterman explained our course of action. He said that we have learned that we cannot kill the Leukemia with chemotherapy but wanted to give Sandy more chemotherapy, not to kill the Leukemia but to hold it down. At the same time he would tapper Sandy off of Tacrolimus gradually to try to create some graft versus host disease. Doctor Letterman said that they couldn't stop the Tacrolimus all of a sudden because she might die from graft versus host disease. When the Tacrolimus was completely out of her body for 4 weeks they planned to infuse some more stem cells they had previously frozen, in hopes that the stem cells would attack any Leukemia that was left and kill it. I asked the doctor what

Sandy's chances were now and he said between 5 and 10%. I didn't tell Sandy that, I just wanted her to know there was still hope. All of this would happen in the hospital so Sandy would be admitted for the 4th. Time that day.

We had to wait in the clinic until they had a hospital bed ready for Sandy and by the time we went to the hospital most of the employees at the clinic had gone home. At about 6:00 P.M. her room was ready and we went to the hospital. I spent the night with Sandy in the hospital that night and the next morning I went back home to check the mail, pay the bills and pet the cats. It was late so I spent the night at home and got up and drove back to the hospital the next morning.

I went back to the hospital as soon as I got back to San Francisco and spent the evening with Sandy. I would spend the days with Sandy at the hospital and go back to the apartment at night to sleep. When Sandy was first admitted to the hospital one of the nurse practioners talked to Sandy about her choices, she could have the treatment or there is hospice if you go home. I thought that strange because I still thought Sandy would be cured. So I got a little angry and said "so what your saying is: Sandy can have the treatment or she can go home and die." I said, "we choose treatment and a chance to live." Then I left the room. A few days later when I went to be with Sandy, she said to me, "Buddy I want to go home even if I have to sneak out of here." I told her that she couldn't go home because her treatment has already started and because of the chemotherapy she would need blood transfusions. When the nurse practioner came in (a different one this time) I said to her, "Sandy wants to go home." She said to me," she can go home now if she wants to." I was taken aback by that statement and told her that I didn't appreciate it. Both of the nurse practioners meant well, they just said it wrong.

I went out to the hall to find the doctor and talk to him. Doctor Garcia was in the hall and I said to him, "I would like to talk to you, when would be a good time?" He said, "how about now, I'm just working my way down the hall." I explained the situation to Doctor Garcia and asked him to explain Sandy's situation and choices to her when he got to her room. I said, "she can't go home in the middle of treatment, she would surely die because she would need blood transfusions." Doctor Garcia didn't say anything to that but I was sure I was right.

I was in Sandy's room when doctor Garcia came in and he did a great job of explaining everything to her. Sandy asked doctor Garcia, "there's still a chance?" He said "yes, but it's small." Sandy asked, "how small." Doctor Garcia told Sandy "5 to 10 %." Sandy seemed glad to hear that she still had a chance to survive.

Sandy had Chemotherapy for seven days this time while the doctors tapered off the Tacrolimus. The Tacrolimus was scheduled to be tapered off completely on December 24th. So we would have to wait until January 24th. For the next infusion of stem cells. The Chemotherapy hit Sandy especially hard this time, she had sores in her mouth and her throat was raw. She couldn't eat so they fed her intravenously. Sandy didn't feel well enough to get up and exercise like she did on her other hospital visits. The nurses took blood tests daily to check her blood counts and liver. Sometimes graft versus host disease attacks a persons liver so they check her liver functions regularly.

Sandy's liver function test came back one day and the numbers were askew. I don't know just what they were, but the nurse practioner said," we need to do a liver biopsy to find out if there is anything wrong with her liver. If there is then we can treat it." She went on to say that the surgical team goes through a vein (kind of like her catheter) and they go down to her liver and take a biopsy. She also said that there was a lot less chance of bleeding doing it that way instead of cutting her open. Before they did the biopsy the doctors ordered blood tests to make sure Sandy's platelet count was high enough to clot and stop the bleeding. The doctors ordered another bag of platelets to make sure her count was high enough. Then the biopsy was performed and the results showed that there was nothing wrong with her liver.

I don't refer to all the doctors by name because there were nine or ten of them that rotated shifts. Sandy said the pain in her throat and mouth was pretty bad so the doctor ordered pain medication for her. The pain medication made Sandy hallucinate and one night after I had gone back to the apartment to sleep, Sandy got out of her bed and walked to the nurses station and wanted to call 911 because she thought they were trying to kill her. The nurses tried to call me to come back to the hospital but they called my home instead of the apartment. The nurses told me about it the next day when I arrived at the hospital. Sandy wanted me to spent nights with her at the hospital after that and I did. The nurses told me that they were going to move Sandy to a room across from the nurses station so they could keep an eye on her but I told them that I would be spending nights there from then on so they kept her in her same room. I went back to the apartment every morning to shower and get something to eat, then I would go back to the hospital to be with my wife.

Our daughter Nicole would call every day to check on her mother and would visit her in the hospital every other day or so, she had time then because she was between semesters. Sandy's mother and brothers and sister would call every couple of days to check on Sandy and see how things were going. My friends Lance and Lane would also call a couple times a week. Our son Michael came to visit his mother on his day off and they had a real nice visit. My friend Lance couldn't get a hold of me because I was at the hospital most of the time and he tried to call the apartment. Lance became worried and when I came home on one of my visits, I had a message from him so I called him to explain. The phone in the apartment didn't have an answering machine and he didn't know the number to Sandy's room.

At Christmas time, Sandy's brother William came to visit Sandy in the hospital and stayed two nights with me in the apartment. The second morning Charles woke up before I did and woke me up and told me that he was going to the hospital to see his sister. I was about an hour behind him getting to the hospital and when I got there, I kissed Sandy as I always do and she said to me, "I can tell you've been smoking again." She was right, I had started smoking again. Maybe Sandy's illness was an excuse, I don't know, but I had a lot of things on my mind. Charles was shocked because he didn't realize that Sandy was in such bad shape even though I called regularly to keep everyone informed. When we got back to the apartment that night he was very emotional and said that he came to give me support but he was the one that needed support. This was before I started spending nights in the hospital with Sandy.

I spent Christmas in the hospital with Sandy and my daughter, Nicole. I bought Sandy a compact disk player and a C. D. So she could listen to her favorite music in the hospital. The next day December 26th. Sandy had to have platelets because her numbers were low, however her body was starting to recover and her numbers were coming up. That day the doctors finished tapering Sandy off the Tacrolimus.

Nicole was going to spend New Year's Eve in the hospital with her mother (she actually stayed three nights) so I used the time to go back home and check the mail, pay the bills and pet the cats. Before I left to go back home Sandy had me go to the mall and buy her four pink boas. Sandy and Nicole were going to decorate her hospital room for New Year's Eve and have a party. When I got back on Jan 1st. They told me what a good time they had. Nicole brought some champagne, even though Sandy couldn't have any, and they watched twelve episodes of (*Sex in the City*). Nicole and I had a good visit with Sandy that day because she was feeling good.

On January 2nd. Sandy coughed up some blood and her mouth was bleeding from the sores, but she was able to eat a little bit of soup. Sandy had platelets today because her counts were low. I went back to the apartment to shower and watch a football game and then I went back to the hospital.

On January 3rd. When I got to the hospital Sandy said that she didn't feel well and would be a grouch. She wanted me to go back to the apartment for the day. After I got back to the apartment I took my shower and watched a move on television. I called her room about 4 P. M. That afternoon and there was no answer and I became worried. I went to the hospital and Sandy wasn't in her room. I asked the nurse where she was and the nurse said that her central venous catheter got infected and they sent her to the operating room to take it out and put a pic line in her arm instead. Sandy's veins were small and it took a nurse that was really good to draw blood or put a pic line in. The nurses at the hospital were really good, they seldom had trouble with her veins. We noticed that her central venous catheter was red for a couple of days and figured it was infected. I stayed in the room and waited for Sandy to come back. When she got back she was fine and I was relieved.

January 4th. Sandy was the same today and the nurse practioner came in to explain that Sandy had to be off Tacrolimus for four weeks before they infused more donor stem cells in hope that the stem cells would attack any Leukemia that was present and kill it. That date being January 24th. Of course we were told this before by the doctor but we often had things explained to us several times by different people.

On January 5th. Sandy had bad stomach pains so the doctors adjusted her medication and ordered a cat scan to see what was going on with her stomach. After they took Sandy out for her cat scan, I went to lunch and bought a paper and a coffee before I went back to Sandy's room. When I got there Sandy was asleep and I kissed her as I always did and she opened her eyes and put her hand on my cheek. She didn't say anything but that image will stay with me forever. It was a touching moment for me. Sandy went back to sleep so I read my paper. Wow! The tsunami death toll reaches 150,000, it's the worst disaster I've ever seen in my lifetime.

The next day Sandy woke up with a headache and her mouth hurt worse than before so she couldn't eat and they were still feeding her intravenously. Sandy still was complaining of stomach pain and the results of the cat scan showed a huge blood clot on Sandy's liver 17 centimeters thick. It bled where they did the biopsy. The nurse practioner explained to us that there was a lining around the liver and the blood clot was between the liver and the lining. She said the blood clot was putting pressure on the wound and the pressure stopped the bleeding. She also explained that Sandy's body would absorb the blood over time and what they were going to do was to control Sandy's pain in the mean time.

Nicole was going to stay with her mother the next night so I drove home to check on things. When I got home I had a message from my friend Lance. I called him back and told him that I was home. Lance and Eloise thought I could use a break and invited me out to dinner at the local steak house. At dinner we talked about Sandy and I proposed a toast, "to Sandy, the most courageous person I know" I said, "next time we go to dinner, Sandy will be with us." I sure felt good to see my friends again and get their support. After dinner they drove me home and the next morning I got up and drove back to San Francisco.

When I got back to the hospital, Sandy was groggy and having trouble with her stomach again. The next day Sandy felt pretty good and I think if it wasn't for the pain they would have released her that day, but I think it'll be a few more days before the doctors get the right combination of pain medications.

All of the nurses liked Sandy, several of them told me that Sandy was their favorite patient. Sandy was so nice to them and always thanked them for their care. One of the nurses told us about her engagement to be married on August 13th. I tried to get her to change it to August 12th. Because that's my birthday but she couldn't.

All of the nurses were great, they only had one or two patients each to take care of so they always responded quickly and did a great job of taking care of Sandy.

16

Looking out the Window

Sandy was released from the hospital on January 11th. A volunteer brought her down in a wheel chair while I went to bring the car around. I parked in front of the hospital and waited for the volunteer to bring her out but he didn't. I looked for her and she was sitting in a chair in the waiting room. She turned around to took at me and I saw her, she had her pretty red coat on and she looked pale, almost white. It's all I could do to hold back the tears, I felt so bad for her and there was nothing I could do. That is another image that will be in my memory forever. I went in and helped her to the car and off to the apartment we went. I'm having trouble writing for any length of time because I can still see her looking out the window. People tell me it's ok to be sad and to greave.

The rest of that day was good for Sandy, she was glad to be out of the hospital and back at the apartment.

Nicole lives close to the apartment and goes to college across the street, so she saw her mother regularly. Nicole was coming to dinner the day after Sandy was released from the hospital and I was going to cook some chicken, rice and vegetables. Nicole told us that a client took her and boss out to a fancy dinner the night before and my dinner was better. That made this novice cook feel pretty good.

Sandy was feeling good all day and even ate her dinner. About an hour after dinner Sandy began having severe stomach pains, so bad that she couldn't hardly stand them. Our instructions were to call the clinic and they would connect us to the doctor on call. I called the clinic right away and the doctor called us back right away. I described Sandy's condition to him and he told us to go to the emergency room and he would meet us there. I explained to the doctor what had been going on with Sandy and they started her on pain medication and took an x-ray. In the emergency room they tried different kinds of pain medication until they got Sandy comfortable. When her pain subsided she went to sleep. The doctor told me that there were no rooms available in the hospital, it was full. Sandy would have to stay in the emergency room until they could find a bed for her.

The doctor also told me that it wouldn't be until the next day. So after Sandy went to sleep I went back to the apartment to sleep. I couldn't sleep and I got up early the next morning and went back to the emergency room. When I got there Sandy was still asleep, so I gave her a kiss and she woke up. Sandy asked me if I had been there all night. I said, "no, I went back to the apartment to sleep and came back early this morning." Sandy had a restful night and didn't know whether I was there or not. The hospital finally had a bed for her that afternoon and they took her up to her home away from home, the 11th. Floor of Long hospital.

Sandy was in the hospital for the fifth time and her condition was worse. Our nurse practioner, Tory, ordered a chest x-ray to see what was causing Sandy's pain and her difficulty breathing. The x-ray showed that Sandy had some liquid on her lungs. Tory told me that they were going to try to draw the liquid out with a needle. Tory would do it and she explained to me that they would go in her back between two ribs. They did the procedure the next day. Sandy never liked me to be in the room when they were doing any kind of procedure so I left for a couple of hours.

The hospital had a family room at the end of the hall with videos, lots of books and a computer. I logged on the computer and found out that I could check my e-mail. That was wonderful because the first time I went home I had over 200 messages. I regularly used the hospital computer after that to keep everyone informed on Sandy's condition.

When I went back to the room, Tory told me that they only got 300 ccs. Of liquid. She said that wasn't very much. As usual Sandy never once complained.

The doctor came in and told me they could try to draw more fluid from Sandy's lungs by inserting a tube in her back and drawing it out that way. The doctor explained that this procedure was safer than a needle because with a needle there was always a chance of puncturing a lung. The hospital scheduled that procedure for the next day. Nicole was there for the procedure and waited with me until it was complete. This time they only got 100 ccs. Of fluid. After Sandy got back to her room the doctor ordered oxygen because Sandy was having a little trouble breathing. The nurses drew blood every day to make sure her blood counts were ok. The doctors ordered more platelets for Sandy and I asked the doctor if that meant that Sandy was bleeding internally and the doctor said, "no, we just want her counts to be higher." The nurse posted the red blood counts, white blood counts, and platelets on a dry erase board in her room. I checked the board every day to see how the blood counts were doing.

Two days later doctor Letterman came in and told us that the Leukemia was back. I asked the doctor, "can we infuse the stem cells now and will they fight the Leukemia?" Doctor Letterman said, "no, there's too many." I said "we're out of treatment options aren't we?" Doctor Letterman said, "yes." Two different doctors pressured us to give them a ressitation or no ressitation decision but we wouldn't.

That was the first time I realized that Sandy was going to die.

Sandy wouldn't sign and advance directive, she just told the doctors that she would leave any decision up to me. Knowing what I know now, we would have gone home after the transplant and not had the rest of the treatment. I just wanted my wife to be cured, I didn't want her to suffer. I loved her so much.

17

A Song

I devoted every minute of my life to Sandy during the last seven months and I felt real good about it. I thought about a song I once herd. It's called "Cats In The Cradle" and the lyrics were by Ugly Kid Joe. I always thought it was a good song that had a lot of truth to it. It goes like this:

Verse 1

My child arrived just the other day
Came to the world in the usual way
But there were planes to catch and bills to pay
He learned to walk while I was away
He was talkin' fore I knew it
And as he grew he said
"I'm gonna be like you, Dad.
You know I'm gonna be like you."

Chorus

And the cat's in the cradle and the silver spoon,
little boy blue and the man 'n the moon
"When you comin' home?"
"Son, I don't know when. We'll get together then.
You know we'll have a good time then."

Verse 2

well, my son turned ten just the other day.
He said, "thanks for the ball, Dad. Come on, let's play.

Could you teach me to throw?"
I said, "Not today. I got a lot to do."
He said, "that's okay." And he walked away and he smiled and he said,
"you know, I'm gonna be like him, yeah.
You know I'm gonna be like him."

Chorus

Verse 3

Well, he came from college just the other day,
So much like a man I just had to say,
"I'm proud of you. Could you sit for a while?"
He shook his head and he said with a smile,
"What I'd really like, Dad, is to borrow the car keys.
See you later. Can I have them please?"

Chorus

Verse 4

I've long since retired, my son's moved away.
I called him up just the other day
"I'd like to see you, if you don't mind."
He said, "I'd love to, Dad, if I could find the time.
You see my new job's a hassle and the kids have the flu,
But it's sure nice talkin' to you."
And as I hung up the phone it occurred to me,
He'd grown up just like me.
My boy was just like me.

Chorus

I think of that song a lot and to me the moral of the story is: Take the time to spend with your loved ones and honor and cherish them because,

Tomorrow never comes.

18

I Think I've Suffered Enough

The doctors were going to keep Sandy in the hospital until they could get her pain under control and then release her. Tory told me that they were going to try a patch and a pill, and that there were different strength patches. They would try different combinations until they found the right formula.

That day in the hospital Sandy said to me, "I think I've suffered enough." and I said, "I think so to.' Sandy said to me, "I just want to go home."

Sandy wanted to die at home so we were trying to find a way to get her home. She was on 100% oxygen because her oxygen saturation level had dropped in to the 80s. I asked the nurse what the oxygen saturation level should be and she told me that an oxygen saturation level of 100 is perfect and it should be in the high 90s. There was no way to set oxygen up in my car so taking her home in the car wouldn't work. My daughter Nicole came up with the solution. She said, "why don't you take her home in an ambulance." One of the nurses coordinates that kind of stuff and she called around to try to find an ambulance company that would go out of town. The nurse found one and made all the arrangements, she also contacted hospice and they would be waiting for us when we got home.

All of the nurses loved Sandy and several of them cam in to her room to give her a hug and tell her goodby. I talked to doctor Letterman and asked him about a chemotherapy pill that kills white blood cells. I thought that might give Sandy a little more quality time at home. Doctor Letterman agreed and wrote the prescription.

Sandy was to go home tomorrow January 22nd. So I went back to the apartment and packed everything up and loaded the car. I then turned in my keys.

I spent the last seven moths waiting for Sandy to get better and it would all be over soon. That night in Sandy's room, Nicole said that she wanted to ride in the ambulance with her mother so she took her car home and I followed and brought her back to the hospital. Nicole arranged to take a weeks vacation so she could be with her mother. When we got back to the hospital the nurse said only one of us could stay in the room with Sandy that night and the other one would have to go down to the lobby and sleep in a chair. Sandy wanted Nicole to stay with her and I said that I would rather go home than sleep in the lobby. So I kissed Sandy and drove home.

It was after 9:00 P.M. by then and I didn't get home until after 1:00 A.M.. I stopped along the way and got a very large coffee to help keep me awake on the drive. When I got home there was a message on my answering machine from the hospice nurse to call her when I got home. Her message said that she didn't mind what time it was when I called. So I called even though it was in the middle of the night. She told me not to fill Sandy's prescriptions that hospice would provide them.

Every time Sandy was released from the hospital we met with the pharmacist and had new prescriptions to pick up. It's a good thing that I told her that I would wait until I got home to pick them up because if I had picked them up in San Francisco, I would have duplicates.

I got up the next morning and went grocery shopping as there was nothing in the house to eat because we emptied out the refrigerator before we left for San Francisco. We told Dana to take what was left when we left. I made arrangements for Dana to be at the house that morning because Apria was going to deliver the oxygen and other supplies while I was out grocery shopping.

Nicole told me that Sandy slept most of the morning but when the ambulance drivers got to the hospital to bring Sandy home, Nicole said, "mom the ambulance is here" and Sandy sat straight up in be and said, "I'm ready." She was so excited about being able to go home after such a long time.

The ambulance arrived at our home at 2:00 P.M. that afternoon and the hospice nurses were there waiting. Sandy wanted to be in her chair instead of bed so the ambulance people brought her in the house and got her comfortable in her chair. The hospice nurses made sure that Sandy was alright and her pain was ok before they left for the day.

Sandy stayed awake for a while and visited with us, she was so glad to be home. She then fell asleep in her chair and I woke her up when it was time to go to bed.

The arrangement was for the hospice nurses to come to the house three times a week but I ended up having them there every day and sometimes several times a day.

January 23rd. Sandy had a good day today. When we got up, I helped her to the living room so she could be in her favorite chair and she visited with us most of the morning and then took a nap. That afternoon our friends Lance and Eloise came to visit with Sandy and she was so happy to see them. She gave each of them a big hug and cried. She visited with them for an hour or so and then they left.

Sandy wanted a root beer float so I went to the store to get some ice cream and root beer. When I got home she was asleep and I didn't want to wake her until it was time for us to go to bed. So she didn't get her root beer float. Maybe she will tomorrow.

January 24th. Sandy was even better today than she was yesterday. Our friends Lane and Clair Yeperson came to visit and Sandy was happy to see them. She gave them both a big hug and they visited for an hour or so. When they left, Sandy fell asleep for a nap. Sandy stayed awake longer today than she did yesterday and wanted a pineapple popsicle. So I went to the store and bought the popsicle and she liked it very much.

She said, "yum."

Our son Michael arrived today to spend some time with his mother. Michael's wife Lona, his daughter Candy and son Hugh came also. Michael's daughter Mary was with her mother and they hadn't arrived yet. They had a nice visit and Sandy was happy to have her family around her.

Our four cats didn't get on Sandy's lap this time, I think they knew something was wrong. Sandy didn't say anything about that but I know she was disappointed.

January 25th. This was Sandy's best day. She got up with me in the morning and stayed up most of the day. She sat in her favorite chair and was glad that her family was with her. I cooked for every one but Sandy didn't eat. We had some strawberries frozen from last summer so I took some of them out of the freezer to thaw and put some banana slices in them for Sandy. After they thawed I gave them to Sandy and she liked them. We had no company today but Sandy's family all called to see how she was doing.

January 26th. I got up early but Sandy was still asleep so I didn't disturb her. I went in the kitchen and fixed breakfast for every one and cleaned up the kitchen. Then I went in to check on Sandy and she was still asleep and was having trouble breathing. I called the hospice nurses to come and check on her. Sandy didn't get out of bed all day. When I told Sandy that I loved her she would answer, "I love you too." and when the kids would talk to her she would always answer them.

January 27th. Sandy didn't get out of bed today either. This time when we talked to her she didn't answer us but I knew she could hear us. Sometimes it sounded like she would try to say something but we couldn't make out what she was saying. I had the hospice nurse out three times today, once was at midnight.

It sounded like she was moaning and I wanted the nurse to adjust her medications so she wouldn't be in pain. Sandy only said one thing that day. All of her family called that day and I would put the phone up to her ear so she could hear them talk to her. When Sandy's mother called she said, "Sandy this is your mother, I love you." and the only thing that Sandy said that day was, "I love you too, mama."

When I went to bed that night Sandy was having a hard time breathing, her eyes were yellow and watering. Her eyes were open most of the day but I'm not sure she saw anything. Sandy was on a pain pump that administered pain medication on a regular basis but she could push the button every ten minutes and get more if she needed. I was going to stay up all night that night and push the button for her if she moaned. I knew she wasn't going to last much longer and it looked like she was suffering so I rolled over and whispered in her ear, "honey, it's time to give up." That was hard for me to do, but I hated to see her suffer and I loved her so much. At midnight it sounded like she was moaning so I got up and called the hospice nurse to come and adjust her medication.

I must have fallen asleep after the hospice nurse left because when I woke up it was 7:30 A.M. and I didn't hear a sound coming from Sandy. I rolled over and Sandy had died, she was cold. The kids knew what had happened because they could hear me crying all the way on the other side of the house. I sobbed, and sobbed and sobbed. I loved her so much. I want her back but I knew that she was gone from my sight forever. I knew she would live in my memory forever. I was so sad. I felt so bad for Sandy. I sat on the edge of my bed for a while with my head in my hands.

I have to stop and dry my eyes.

After I sat on the edge of my bed for some time, I got up and went to the living room to tell the kids what had happened. They already knew. Neither Michael, nor Nicole said anything, they just stared into space and their eyes were watering. They both were silent for a while but I knew how much they were hurting inside. We gave each other a hug. I asked my son Michael to call Hospice and told them that they would take care of everything. We didn't talk while we were waiting for the hospice nurse to come, we just sat around in a trance.

It didn't take long for the nurse to arrive. The hospice nurse and my daughter Nicole changed Sandy into some nice clothes and the nurse called the mortuary.

After the mortuary came and took Sandy to the funeral home, we didn't do anything the rest of the day. We just sat around and I paced a lot.

19

Life After Death

My son Michael and my daughter, Nicole stayed with me for a few days after Sandy died and went with me to make the funeral arrangements. I'm glad they did because it made taking care of the arrangements easier.

Sandy told me one time that she didn't want a funeral when she died but I wanted it to honor her. Sandy's side of the family lived out of town so we set the date on a Saturday so they could all come. I notified all of her family and our friends of the date and time of the funeral ahead of time so they could arrange their schedules.

The day of the funeral came and I was a bit nervous, I don't know why, I just was. Every one came to honor Sandy and I was pleased to see everyone there. After the services everyone came to my house for a reception and stayed for a couple of hours. Sandy's mother, Elaine said that it was the best funeral she had ever been to.

Some of the people brought food and flowers. One of my friends brought some plastic containers and froze the food that was left so I could have some quick freezer meals when I didn't feel like cooking. Every one helped to clean up the house before they left, which was much appreciated.

I've lost my mother (of diabetes), my father (heart attack), my older brother (of heart failure), and now my wife. For me losing my life long partner was a lot worse than losing either of my parents or my brother. When people that have lost a parent said to me, "I know how you feel." They really don't.

Michael and Nicole stayed until the next day and then had to go home on Sunday.

After everyone had left, I looked around and realized for the first time that I was all alone.

For the first few weeks after Sandy's death, I stayed busy working in the yard. The weeds had taken over all of the flower beds and planting areas. We had built a gravel path around the putting green and it took me three days just to pull all of the weeds out of the path.

One day I was pulling weeds from under a Japanese Maple tree that Sandy and I planted. Sandy's brother Sparky bought the tree for us and we planted it on what would have been my older brothers 60th. Birthday. I started thinking of Sandy and the recent events and I started crying. I said out loud," Honey, I'm trying. I'm trying." I was doing the gardening and have never done it before. Sandy always did all the gardening.

Even though I tried to stay busy, I couldn't sleep at night. The events of the last eight months of Sandy's life kept swirling around in my head and I couldn't shut my mind off. I got up one night around 3:00 A.M. and began to write everything down. I would sit in my office in my underwear and write. As I write now it's 3:30 A.M. on a Saturday morning and I'm in my underwear again. I write for a while and it brings back the memories and the pain so I have to stop every so often and dry my eyes. After I finished writing all I could remember down, I was able to sleep most of the time.

After I finished with the yard work, I felt lost. I didn't know what to do with myself. I do play golf with my friends once a week, but that leaves six other days to fill in. My son and daughter call me a couple of times a week to see if I'm alright. They're worried about me. Bless their hearts.

The hospice councilor has called me several times to see how I was doing and told me about a free group session for people that have lost loved ones and thought I might like to attend. I never did go to any of these sessions, but it is nice to know there is help out there if a person needs help.

My friends suggested joining a health club but I just don't feel like it right now. Lance told me that every day would get a little bit better. Wrong. What I can tell you is that the healing process is a lot slower than that. I would say that every month is a little bit better than the last.

My friends suggested that I make lists for myself. I do that and I do some of the things on the list, but never seem to be able to make myself finish. I know that eventually I will get in some sort of a routine, I just don't know how long it will take.

When I go out in the yard to do the watering, I can see that I have neglected some of the yard work. Will I do it? I don't know. I'll probably get around to it one of these days.

My daughter Nicole came to visit me for a couple of days. We went to a movie and just hung out together. When she had to leave to go back home she said to me, "you're doing just fine." I hated to say goodby to her but she had to get back home and back to work again.

I did have a yard sale and sold some of Sandy's stuff and some things that I no longer wanted. It was hard to go through her things and I still have a lot to go through. Her purse is still hanging on our bedroom door and her clothes are still in our closet. The picture of Sandy and I that's in this book is on a night stand by our sofa. I give her a kiss every night when I go to bed. Sandy's ashes are on the headboard of our bed and there they will stay.

The hardest day for me so far was June 22,2005, it would have been Sandy's 56th. birthday. When I got up that morning I told myself that I was going to finish building the fence for her birthday and I did finish. Happy Birthday Sandy.

That night my friends Lance and Eloise Butterman invited my over for dinner. They knew what a special day June 22nd. was. Lance barbequed a london broil steak and we had a salad and corn on the cob. We ate out on the back patio that is shaded by an arbor. In the backyard they have a pool with a waterfall. It's very warm that time of year in Redding and they eat outside a lot. Lance has finished landscaping his backyard and it's beautiful. He did a good job. The landscaping is pleasing to the eye and the flowers were in full bloom. The smell of the fresh air and the flowers made the dining experience a very pleasant one.

Lane and Clair Yeperson call me from time to time and check on me to see if I'm doing alright. Sometimes we get together and Lane will cook dinner. I think I'm lucky to have two best friends.

It's been six months now since Sandy died and I think I'm doing fine despite losing my life long companion and my best friend. It's hard for me to explain what and how I feel. I've used words like lost, in a trance and not knowing what to do with myself. I do know that I'm going to be alright, it might take some time but I'll be fine. Some days I care and some days I don't. Some times I wish the pain would go away and sometimes I realize that the pain is evidence of how much I loved and cared for my wife and best friend.

Nicole graduated from San Francisco State University on May 28th, 2005. Four months to the day since Sandy died. It was a very happy and sad day for me. Sandy was looking forward to seeing Nicole graduate and she didn't live long enough so I went by myself. I met Nicole after the ceremony and took her out to dinner. I promised her a trip to Australia for her graduation present. Nicole is so excited about going and it gives me something to look forward to.

I don't like to stay home all day so sometimes I just go for a drive down the freeway and back. Driving seems to allow me to clear my head, think things out, and contemplate what lies ahead for me. I don't know what that is yet, but I'm sure it will come in time.

I'm not ready for a lady friend yet, that time might or might not come. I'm not in a hurry though, I have all the time in the world. For now my heart still belongs to Sandy.

As I said, I wrote all of this down for therapy for myself and then I thought, if I could help just one person get through a tragedy like this maybe I should publish the story.

Unfortunately half of us that are married are eventually going to have to deal with the death of our spouse.

A few days before Sandy died the hospice nurse gave me a pamphlet to read titled "gone from my sight" and inside was the following quote:

I am standing upon the seashore. A ship at me side spreads her white sails to the morning breeze and starts for the blue ocean. She is an object of beauty and strength. I stand and watch her until at length she hangs like a speck of white cloud just where the sea and sky come to mingle with each other.

Then someone at my side says: "There, she is gone!"

"Gone where?"

Gone from my sight. That is all. She is just as large in mast and hull and spar as she was when she left my side and she is just as able to bear her load of living freight to her destined port.

Her diminished size is in me, not in her. And just at the moment when someone at my side says: "There, she is gone!" there are other eyes watching her coming, and other voices ready to take up the glad shout: "Here she comes!:

and that is dying.

Henry Van Dyke

978-0-595-36293-6
0-595-36293-1

www.ingramcontent.com/pod-product-compliance
Lightning Source LLC
Chambersburg PA
CBHW020336290526
45785CB00005B/2051

* 9 780595 362936 *